KILLER
DOCTORS

KILLER DOCTORS

COLIN EVANS

BERKLEY BOOKS, NEW YORK

THE BERKLEY PUBLISHING GROUP
Published by the Penguin Group
Penguin Group (USA) Inc.
375 Hudson Street, New York, New York 10014, USA
Penguin Group (Canada), 90 Eglinton Avenue East, Suite 700, Toronto, Ontario M4P 2Y3, Canada
(a division of Pearson Penguin Canada Inc.)
Penguin Books Ltd., 80 Strand, London WC2R 0RL, England
Penguin Group Ireland. 25 St. Stephen's Green, Dublin 2, Ireland (a division of Penguin Books Ltd.)
Penguin Group (Australia), 250 Camberwell Road, Camberwell, Victoria 3124, Australia
(a division of Pearson Australia Group Pty. Ltd.)
Penguin Books India Pvt. Ltd., 11 Community Centre, Panchsheel Park, New Delhi 110 017, India
Penguin Group (NZ), 67 Apollo Drive, Rosedale, North Shore 0745, Auckland, New Zealand
(a division of Pearson New Zealand Ltd.)
Penguin Books (South Africa) (Pty.) Ltd., 24 Sturdee Avenue, Rosebank, Johannesburg 2196,
South Africa

Penguin Books Ltd., Registered Offices: 80 Strand, London WC2R 0RL, England

KILLER DOCTORS

A Berkley Book / published by arrangement with the author

PRINTING HISTORY
First published in Great Britain by Michael O'Mara Books Limited / 1993
Berkley mass-market edition / June 2007

Copyright © 1993, 2007 by Colin Evans
Book design by Kristin del Rosario

ISBN: 978-0-425-21601-9

BERKLEY®
Berkley Books are published by The Berkley Publishing Group,
a division of Penguin Group (USA) Inc.,
375 Hudson Street, New York, New York 10014.
BERKLEY is a registered trademark of Penguin Group (USA) Inc.
The "B" design is a trademark belonging to Penguin Group (USA) Inc.

PRINTED IN THE UNITED STATES OF AMERICA

10 9 8 7 6 5 4 3 2 1

Acknowledgments

I am deeply indebted to the following people and organizations: Wayne T. Seay, chief of detectives, Nassau County Police Department; Tina Vicini, Chicago Police Department; Gerard J. Sciaraffa, Circuit Court of Cook County, Illinois; Lieutenant Dennis Bingheim and Sergeant John Summers of the Quincy, Illinois, police department; Chief Terrence M. Cunningham and Detective Peter L. McLaughlin of the Wellesley Police Department, Massachusetts; Samantha Mandor at Berkley; David Andersen; and Greg Manning. A very special thank-you to Ed Knappman and everyone at New England Publishing Associates.

Research staff at the New York Public Library, National Archives, Library of Congress, Broward County Library in Florida, the New York State Archives, the British Library, and the British Newspaper Library at Colindale, London, all provided unstinting and selfless assistance.

The usual caveat applies: while all of these people contributed so much to this book, the responsibility for any errors is mine alone.

Contents

1. A WOMAN SCORNED

Sex, jealousy, murder and revenge—the staples of classic drama. Shakespeare fashioned a masterpiece from such stuff and called it *Othello*. Three and a half centuries later, in 1966, nothing much had changed except that, on this occasion, the drama was played out in two courtrooms, the press screamed "Love Triangle Slaying!" and the leading player was not a Moorish general but a thirty-four-year-old, darkly handsome doctor with an angular smile. He did have a stagey ring to his name, though—Carl Anthony Coppolino.

He grew up the son of a barber in Brooklyn, New York. The Coppolinos were typical of the neighborhood they lived in—never quite enough money at the end of the week for extras, but no great shortages either. Just an average, everyday family. Except that Carl was far from being the average kid. In the first place he was bright, very bright; secondly, his ambition was ruthless and knew no bounds. He worked hard at school, saved up his allowance and secured a place at Fordham University where he studied medicine. On campus he kept himself to himself, even though his lean features drew plenty of admiring glances from the coeds. He seemed preoccupied with his work and, anyway, he was already dating seriously.

Carmela Musetto first met Coppolino in 1952 when she was a pre-med student at Trinity College in Washington DC. She was as cute as a button and the two hit it off right away, despite big differences in their backgrounds. Whereas Coppolino constantly had to struggle to meet costly tuition fees, Carmela's father, a successful physician, was always on call whenever his daughter needed a helping financial hand. In 1956 Carmela joined Coppolino at the Downstate Medical Center. That same year she also became his bride.

The arrival of a baby daughter, Monica, sent Coppolino's perpetual money problems into a serious tailspin. Only a bailout from Carmela's father enabled him to finish his studies and qualify as an MD. After graduation both he and his wife did their internships at the Methodist Hospital in Brooklyn. From there, Carmela decided against regular practice and took a position as a research physician with a large pharmaceutical firm, while Coppolino became staff anesthesiologist at Riverview Hospital in Red Bank, New Jersey.

It was around this time that Coppolino first became interested in hypnosis. In the fifties hypnosis was just beginning to gain credibility as a useful medical tool. Coppolino was quick to realize its possibilities and soon became a skilled practitioner. He would induce patients to relax before surgery and also assist them in dealing with postoperative discomfort. Aside from the obvious medical benefits, Coppolino also saw hypnosis as a handy means of substantially boosting his income. He began treating patients at home, helping to rid them of undesirable habits or to alleviate pain. He prospered, but still the extra money wasn't enough; he kept pushing for more. At Riverview his reputation was that of a whiner, forever carping about the paltry salary paid to anesthesiologists. As his greed worsened, so did his temper. Inexorably, the darker side of Carl Coppolino's nature began to surface.

He became obsessive about one of the staff nurses, constantly bitching to his colleagues that she was receiving money which rightfully should have gone to them. It was an extraordinary accusation to make, entirely without foundation, but Coppolino was unrelenting. Soon the nurse was on the receiving end of a barrage of abusive letters and anonymous phone calls, all telling her to quit the hospital— or else. At first she shrugged off the threats but, as their intensity grew so did her apprehension and she contacted the authorities. An FBI agent visited the hospital. He speedily concluded that the virulent campaign had its origins inside the hospital. His suspicions were aroused by a room which housed several typewriters. Forensic tests proved that at least some of the threatening letters had been written on these very machines. Next, he checked out who used the room most often. The name of Dr. Carl Coppolino kept cropping up. Coppolino's animosity toward the nurse was remembered and led to a confrontation. He made no great pretense of denying anything, and the hospital, anxious to avoid scandal, allowed him to resign quietly without pressing any charges.

Coppolino explained away the resignation to acquaintances as medically caused, the result of a persistent heart condition. As if to prove the point he filed a claim with his insurance company for disability benefits. It was later learned that he had dosed himself with digitalis which produces abnormal patterns in electrocardiograms, irregularities easily mistaken for heart disease. Grudgingly, the insurance company began paying him $1,500 a month. Added to this, his wife's annual salary of $15,000 was enough for Dr. Carl Coppolino to retire on. Best of all, he was still only thirty years old.

Coppolino stayed in his split-level home in the fashionable Fox Run district of Middletown, New Jersey, and settled down to the life of an aspiring writer. Success came soon. He published a book entitled *The Practice of Hypnosis in Anesthesiology*, quickly followed by *Freedom from Fat*. At this point Carl Coppolino might have faded into relative obscurity as a mildly successful author and unsuspected insurance fraud. That he did not is due entirely to the fact that, one afternoon, Carmela threw a party for her newborn daughter, Lisa. She invited several of the neighbors. Among those present was a glamorous forty-eight-year-old housewife, Marjorie Farber.

Marjorie and her husband, Colonel William Farber, recently retired after a long and distinguished military career, were prominent local socialites. Together they took the Coppolinos under their wing. During the day Marge would ferry the ailing Carl to libraries and other places of interest to a writer intent on research. In the course of these excursions Coppolino enlarged upon his heart complaint, telling Marge that the doctors had only given him another five years to live. Marge's sympathy was aroused. She and her husband resolved to do what they could.

On the surface the two families seemed unlikely companions—the Coppolinos were almost two decades younger—but Marjorie Farber more than made up for any disparity in their ages by demonstrating the verve and vivacity of a woman half her years. She was uncommonly attractive. With her voluptuous figure, she could still fill out a bikini and she could still turn heads. Unfortunately, just about the only thing Marge couldn't do was stop smoking. At Carmela's prompting she turned to Carl. He listened sympathetically and explained how a course of hypnotic suggestion might help. On February 4, 1963, he went to the Farber home and began treatment. It worked. Marge didn't touch another cigarette for two years. But, as one vice disappeared, so another took its place.

With their respective spouses out at work—ironically, William had taken employment with an insurance firm— days at Fox Run for the couple were long and blessedly free from interruption. As the hypnosis sessions developed that first week, Marge felt her resistance dwindle. She later described an atmosphere heavily charged with carnal expectation. It was hardly surprising; both she and Carl were highly sexed. Perhaps fearful of Coppolino's alleged heart condition, Marge held off as best she could. But she soon succumbed to his persistent advances. From that moment on, Carl and Marge made love at every available opportunity.

If Carmela suspected anything she never said, not even when ailing Carl announced a forthcoming holiday in Florida. The warmer weather, he felt, would improve his health. Unable to go herself, Carmela expressed delight when Marge volunteered to go along to "take care of him."

William Farber's attitude was less conciliatory. Already suspicious, he argued bitterly that it would make him look foolish in the community if his wife were to fly off with another woman's husband. But Marge was nothing if not persuasive and wore down his objections, one by one, until finally she gained his approval.

With the gossipy tongues of Fox Run rattling in their ears, patient and nurse headed for Florida.

If Marjorie Farber's later claims are to be believed then there was very little evidence of Carl Coppolino's "coronary insufficiency" during this ten-day jaunt to Miami Beach. "We had intercourse at least three times a day; I don't know how he did it." But William Farber clearly did, and when these trips began almost to stumble over each other in their frequency, his suspicions became more vocal and virulent.

This suited Marge; marital unrest was just the ticket for what she and Coppolino had in mind. While in Miami Beach, Coppolino had drawn up a "love plan," which laid down explicit guidelines for the future conduct of their affair. First and foremost was his jealous insistence that Marge not sleep with her husband. Coppolino wanted them to live as "brother and sister." Failing that, he told Marge, "either get an annulment or a divorce."

It took her a month, but Marge was able to dislodge William Farber from her bedroom. Their rows became increasingly bitter. Coppolino didn't mind. The initial stage of his "love plan" had worked. Now it was time for stage two.

On the evening of July 30, 1963, the Coppolinos were at home when the telephone rang. It was Marge, on the verge of panic. Apparently one of her daughters had entered their bedroom and found William Farber unconscious. Unable to waken him, the girl ran to her mother, crying, "Daddy looks awful funny." Marge pleaded for Carl to come over right away.

Coppolino did some quick thinking. If the insurance company caught him practicing medicine it would mean the end of his disability benefit; better for Carmela to go over alone. He did mention, though, that Farber had suffered convulsions the day previously, the kind that often precede a heart attack.

Carmela found William Farber dead in the bedroom.

Apart from being "all blue down one side," there was no outward sign of distress to the body. At Carl's urging, she dutifully signed the death certificate, citing "coronary thrombosis" as the cause. Farber's body was transferred to the National Cemetery in Arlington, Virginia, where he was buried with full military honours. Marge attended the funeral with Carmela. Carl decided to stay at home. The following weekend he and Marge went to Atlantic City, alone.

Things soon quieted down in Fox Run. Carl resumed his writing and published two more books. Carmela went back to the high-paying pharmaceutical firm. Both remained on the best of terms with Marjorie Farber. Especially Carl. Their affair bubbled along for another eighteen months, then abruptly cooled as Carl began to tire of the amorous widow's attentions. She was getting too pushy. Respite came in April 1965 when Carmela took six months' severance pay from her pharmaceutical job. She and Carl sold their New Jersey home and moved to Florida, where they bought a house on ritzy Longboat Key, an exclusive island retreat just across the bay from Sarasota. At last Coppolino had the monkey off his back.

It should have been the best of times for the young married couple and their two daughters, but calamity was just around the corner. Carmela failed the Florida medical examination. This meant that she could not practice in the state. Worse, it meant that Carl would no longer have her income to rely on. Adding to Coppolino's distress, his insurance company was beginning to question the veracity of his alleged disability, putting his monthly benefit check in grave jeopardy. With Carmela's severance pay almost gone, and staring financial disaster right in the face, Coppolino's response was predictable. He met a wealthy divorcée named Mary Gibson at the Maxwell Bridge Studio and began dating her with an eye to future marriage.

But he had reckoned without the tenacity of his erstwhile lover, Marjorie Farber.

She had also moved to Longboat Key, bought some land near the Coppolinos, and had a house built. Furthermore, she was fully expecting to take up where she and Carl had left off. It did not work out that way. Instead, she caught the romantic doctor and his new "bridge partner" together in a parked car, and they didn't appear to be discussing slams and bids. Furious, Marge stormed off to Carmela and told her just what was going on. Coppolino owned up to the affair and requested a divorce. Carmela, a devout Catholic, turned him down cold. Coppolino decided that something had to be done.

At 6 AM August 28, 1965, the Coppolino family physician, Dr. Juliette Karow, was aroused from her bed by a phone call. Short, fortyish and very precise in her manner, Dr. Karow listened to an obviously distraught Carl Coppolino explain how he had just found his wife dead, ostensibly the victim of a heart attack. Karow was puzzled—young women in their thirties rarely suffer coronary failure and Carmela had always seemed in the best of health—but she had no reason to disbelieve Coppolino, especially when he said that Carmela had been complaining of chest pains the night before but pooh-poohed his suggestion that they call a doctor.

Twenty minutes later Karow arrived at the imposing house in Bowsprit Lane. Coppolino met her at the door and showed her into the bedroom. Carmela Coppolino was clearly dead. Karow found no vital signs at all. But she was also deeply troubled. The position of the body seemed unnatural. Carmela lay on her right side, with her right arm tucked beneath her. Karow would have expected to find the hand swollen. It was not. Also, lividity—the tendency of blood to drain to the lowest reaches of the body—did not seem consistent. Neither was the bedding rumpled. On the contrary, it seemed remarkably in place. Everything had the appearance of having been staged.

Karow kept her suspicions to herself and carried on with the examination. Coppolino hovered nearby. At one point Karow saw him clutching at his chest. She also saw him taking some white pills. He shrugged off her caution to be careful, saying that he knew what he was doing. Dr. Karow continued. Ultimately she signed a death certificate, citing "coronary occlusion," and passed her findings to the Sarasota County Medical Examiner who decided that there were no grounds for a postmortem.

Carmela's body was shipped back to her family in New Jersey for burial. Heartbroken, Carl couldn't bring himself to attend to any of the funeral arrangements. He left everything in the hands of relatives. Too upset, he said. Just forty-one days later the grieving widower put his misery behind him and married Mary Gibson. One of his neighbors, George Thomson, was surprised that Coppolino had waited that long. Thomson later testified that, on August 29, just one day after Carmela's death, Coppolino had told him "that he thought it best if he married right away."

Marjorie Farber took the news of Coppolino's marriage badly. With no one to share her bed at night she had plenty of time to brood. In her eyes, she had been duped by Coppolino. He had strung her along and then ditched her for another, younger woman. Such humiliation was unbearable. Resentment and rage festered in her breast but there was something else as well, a dreadful, overwhelming sense of guilt. After weeks of indecision Marjorie

Farber decided to come clean. She went to Dr. Juliette Karow and unburdened her soul.

It was a sensational tale, one that would fill front pages across America for months—how she had been hypnotized into attempting murder and, when that had failed, stood by, a helpless onlooker, as her husband was smothered to death by Dr. Carl Coppolino.

According to Marjorie's subsequent trial testimony, she told an incredulous Karow that she had been under Coppolino's spell ever since he had first hypnotized her to get rid of her smoking habit. She was powerless to deny him anything, especially when he told her repeatedly, "that bastard has got to go," meaning William Farber. Marge went on to explain how Coppolino had given her a syringe filled with some deadly solution and instructions to inject Farber when he was asleep. At the last moment her nerve failed but not before she had injected a minute amount of the fluid into Farber's leg. When he became ill she summoned Coppolino to the house. He first administered a sedative, then attempted to resolve the dangerous situation by wrapping a plastic bag around Farber's head. As the two men struggled, Marge begged Coppolino to stop. He did so. As Farber recovered, he groggily ordered Coppolino from the house. The homicidal doctor retaliated by stuffing a pillow into Farber's face. And this time Coppolino did not stop; he pressed with all his might. Added insurance came in the form of manual strangulation when Marge wasn't watching. In a matter of seconds, William Farber lay dead on the bed.

Not unnaturally, Dr. Karow was stunned by these revelations and insisted that Marjorie repeat her story to a local clergyman. He, in turn, advised them to contact the FBI, which passed the enquiry to the Sarasota County Sheriff's department. Ordinarily, jilted lovers receive a skeptical hearing from any arm of the law but, in this instance, there was corroborating suspicion. Carmela's father, Carmelo Musetto, had moved to Sarasota to be near his grandchildren. But there was something troubling him. He recalled a telephone conversation with Coppolino in which the bereaved husband stated that Dr. Karow's diagnosis of "coronary occlusion" had been confirmed by autopsy. Mr. Musetto, however, knew that no autopsy had taken place; he had been told as much by the funeral director. When questioned by the police as to why he had not come forward sooner, the poor man confessed to being scared that Coppolino would prevent him from seeing his grandchildren. He later testified: "I was lost. I was a lost man."

A discreet investigation began. It spread to New Jersey where authorities uncovered the disturbing fact that Carmela had not attended William Farber during his illness, as she claimed, but was instead at work. Further inquiries revealed that Coppolino had increased the life insurance on Carmela shortly before her death to a sum of $65,000. He had already received $40,000, but one of the insurance companies was refusing to pay up, claiming that Coppolino had misrepresented the state of Carmela's health at the time of the proposal. Coppolino, nothing if not confident, began legal proceedings.

But the net was drawing in. Details of that ugly incident with the nurse at Riverview Hospital all those years before came to light. Investigators thought it clearly demonstrated the vicious side of Carl Coppolino. Authorities in Florida and New Jersey felt they had sufficient grounds to order the exhumation of both bodies. The autopsies were carried out by Dr. Milton Helpern, New York's celebrated chief medical examiner. He found nothing wrong with William Farber's heart but a whole lot wrong with his neck. The cricoid cartilage was fractured in two places. In plain language, the colonel had been strangled.

Next, Helpern switched his attention to the body of Carmela Coppolino. Here, his task proved more difficult. Once again he ruled out any coronary disease; Carmela's heart was in fine shape. Unfortunately for Helpern, so was everything else. Even when he discovered an almost invisible hypodermic puncture mark on Carmela's left buttock it did not help. A battery of forensic tests revealed nothing. It was beginning to look very much as if the perfect murder had taken place.

Helpern, veteran of over 20,000 autopsies, was baffled. At this point frustration set in and speculation took over. Helpern considered Coppolino's former profession and asked himself the question—what type of drug would an anesthesiologist have access to in his work that might cause untraceable death? He was irresistibly drawn to an artificial form of curare called succinylcholine chloride.

The scenario that Helpern worked up was horrific. Succinylcholine chloride causes complete muscular paralysis but does not induce unconsciousness: this meant that, as Carmela's lungs shut down and refused to function, she would have been fully aware of what was happening to her and totally incapable of doing anything about it. A crueler form of suffocation is beyond imagination. Every textbook said that the drug was undetectable. Experts knew that it broke down into other chemicals in the body, but what those chemicals were no one had been able to establish. It was time to call in the poison specialists.

Dr. Charles Umberger, chief of the medical examiner's toxicological department, listened to Helpern's problem and promised to work on it. What followed was truly bizarre. In order to replicate as closely as possible the condition of Carmela Coppolino's body at the time of autopsy,

Umberger injected rabbits and frogs with a solution of succinylcholine chloride, then buried the carcasses and waited to see what would happen. It took six months of painstaking experimentation, but eventually he was able positively to identify the chemicals (and their quantities) that succinylcholine chloride degrades to in the body.

The outcome of this forensic wizardry was the discovery of an excessive amount of succinic acid in Carmela's brain—definite proof that she had received an intravenous injection of succinylcholine chloride sometime before her death. When police pursued this lead they learned that, before Carmela's death, Coppolino had obtained considerable amounts of succinylcholine chloride from a pharmaceutical colleague, explaining that he wished to conduct some experiments on cats. Armed with this knowledge, the Florida State attorney, Frank Schaub, felt confident enough to put his case to a grand jury. They immediately returned an indictment against Coppolino, charging him with the murder of his wife.

Coppolino was at his home on Longboat Key when the police showed up to arrest him. As they led him away he seemed in a state of shock. An already bleak situation worsened considerably when New Jersey announced that Coppolino would also be charged for the death of William Farber. The doctor vociferously protested his innocence, claiming that Marjorie Farber was a compulsive liar out to frame him. But with the evidence stacking up against him, Coppolino did the smartest thing possible: he hired the top criminal defense lawyer in America.

F. Lee Bailey was then at the peak of his celebrity. Only a month before, the newspapers had been full of his exploits in securing a retrial for Sam Sheppard, another physician accused of wife-murder. Flamboyant and bull-necked, Bailey knew all the tricks: when to wheedle, when to bully, when to throw feints, when to quit—the consummate courtroom performer. He moved promptly for a dismissal of both indictments. When this motion was denied he tried another tack—playing one state off against the other.

Because of all the political brownie points that would accrue to whichever prosecutor's office nailed Coppolino, a bitter rivalry had broken out between New Jersey and Florida for the right to try him. As things stood, Florida was the hot favorite since it already had Coppolino under lock and key. Schaub clearly thought so and confidently began preparing his prosecution. Then Florida Governor Hayden Burns inexplicably ordered the extradition of Coppolino to New Jersey.

It was an extraordinary decision, one that Bailey exploited unmercifully, trumpeting that the volte-face clearly demonstrated the weakness of the Florida case. But deep down Bailey was worried. Beneath the brash exterior ticked a shrewd legal brain. He would have preferred to face the Florida charge first; the evidence there was all circumstantial. In New Jersey he had to contend with an eyewitness and evidence of manual strangulation. Even so, Bailey boasted to a couple newsmen: "If I can't win this one, I'll pull down my shingle."

After much legal fencing, the trial began on December 5, 1966. A swarm of journalists descended on the Monmouth County courthouse from all across the nation and even abroad; interest was at a fever pitch. No one came away disappointed.

From the prosecution's opening address, it was evident that their entire case hinged on the testimony of two key witnesses, Marjorie Farber and Dr. Milton Helpern. What they had to say could send Coppolino to the electric chair. Prosecutor Vincent Keuper concluded by loftily declaring that Coppolino had broken not only the commandment "Thou shalt not covet thy neighbor's wife," but also "Thou shalt not covet thy neighbor's life." Unwittingly, with this heavy-handed remark, Keuper set the tone for the whole trial. Morals as much as facts would decide the issue and, in some cases, overshadow them.

Bailey, in his opening statement, came out firing. His only hope lay in totally discrediting Marjorie Farber's character. Break her testimony and Helpern's words would fall on deaf ears; he was certain of that. Bailey unleashed a ringing indictment. "This woman," he told the jury, "drips with venom on the inside, and I hope before we are through you will see it drip on the outside. She wants this man so badly that she would sit on his lap in the electric chair while somebody pulled the switch, just to make sure that he dies. This is not a murder case at all. This is monumental and shameful proof that hell hath no fury like a woman scorned."

When Bailey sat down, the battle lines had been drawn. The watching reporters eagerly sharpened their pencils. For once they had a case that showed every sign of living up to its pretrial publicity. They did not have long to wait. The prosecution called its first witness.

Marjorie Farber.

A buzz filled the courtroom. Everyone craned for a better glimpse of this siren who had ensnared a man eighteen years her junior. But anyone expecting a hip-swinging sex bomb was in for a bitter disappointment. Under guidance from counsel, Marge came dressed in a demure navy-blue outfit, with matching shoes and bag. Completing the unlikely ensemble was a pair of crisp white gloves. One journalist muttered that she must have gotten the days mixed up; she looked ready for Sunday church.

Marge took the stand and primly began her testimony.

She repeated her version of the grisly murder scene and her
own role in it, a helpless pawn in the evil doctor's clutches.
All her free will was destroyed, said Marge; just being in
the same room as Coppolino reduced her to weak-kneed
compliance. Glancing across at the defendant, Marge
added a little verisimilitude to her claim by suddenly
swooning in the witness box. Someone rushed forward
with smelling salts to revive her. Old courtroom hands
thought the scene a touch overdone and nodded sagely.
What the implacable Coppolino thought is anybody's
guess. By the conclusion of her testimony Marjorie Farber
had painted such a black case against the defendant that
she must have felt confident of her ability to face even F.
Lee Bailey. If so, her confidence was gravely misplaced.
What followed was brutal and at times belligerent; it also
remains a classic of legal cross-examination.

Bailey, a pugnacious, stocky man, bulled into her. There
had been no murder at all; everything she said had been a
lie, a figment of Marjorie Farber's malicious imagination,
instigated by an evil desire for revenge on the man who
had ditched her. Wasn't that right? Against a torrent of
prosecution objections Bailey went for the kill: "This
whole story is a cock-and-bull story, isn't it?"

Sustained.

"Didn't you make this all up, Mrs. Farber?"

Sustained.

"Did you fabricate this story?"

Sustained.

Shifting tactics, Bailey went on to ridicule Marge's
claim of having been an unwilling but helpless participant
in the murder, saying he would produce medical testimony
to prove such obeisance impossible. Another thing, said
Bailey: what possible motive could Coppolino have in
killing her husband? He was already taking Marge to his

bed. They had a nice cozy arrangement. Why should Coppolino jeopardize all that? In pursuing this line of attack, Bailey went out on a limb. Many might have considered an attractive, malleable widow with a $50,000 house sufficient motive for an out-of-work doctor to kill for, but the prosecution let this opportunity slide.

Marjorie Farber persisted in her claims but Bailey kept hacking away, constantly reminding the jury of her adulterous and jealous behavior and, most of all, of her age. "This fifty-two-year-old woman" was a repeated theme to the jury, as if this were reason enough to explain Marge's vitriolic accusations. It was crude and it was cruel but it was also effective. Imperceptibly, the mood of the court swung against Marge. For two days her ordeal lasted. At the end of it all Marjorie Farber limped from the stand, her credibility in tatters.

She was replaced by Dr. Milton Helpern, a witness made of much sterner stuff. His evidence was professionally given but even this seasoned courtroom veteran reeled under the Bailey bludgeon. The major points of contention were whether William Farber had suffered from heart disease, and if the cricoid fracture had occurred before or after death. Helpern was emphatic on both issues, although Bailey drew from him the grudging admission that there was no bruising about the neck as would normally have been present if strangulation had taken place. Warming to his theme, Bailey went on to suggest that rough handling of the body during disinterment, in particular a clumsy grave digger's shovel, had caused the cricoid fracture. Helpern scoffed at such an idea. But Bailey had his own expert witnesses and they thought otherwise.

Doctors Joseph Spelman and Richard Ford, both experienced medical examiners, expressed the view that not only was the cricoid fracture caused after death but that

Farber's heart showed clear signs of advanced coronary disease, certainly enough to have killed him.

With the verdict still very much up in the air Bailey called his star witness—Carl Anthony Coppolino.

Always the highpoint of any murder trial is that moment when the defendant takes the stand. He or she is not obliged to do so by law, and most would be better off if they didn't, but Carl Coppolino was no ordinary defendant. Slim and sleekly groomed, the doctor answered his accusers well and he answered them with no noticeable guile. Not once was the prosecution able to shake him from his assertion of having attended William Farber the day before his death for chest pains, and recommending that he should go immediately into the hospital for treatment. Coppolino came across as confident without seeming cocky, helpful but not obsequious. All things considered, it was a very strong showing.

Trial Judge Elvin R. Simmill, in his final summing up, commented on the vast array of conflicting medical evidence and reminded the jury that they must be satisfied of Coppolino's guilt "beyond a reasonable doubt." It was an admonition that the jury took to heart. After deliberating for less than five hours they returned a verdict of not guilty.

Among the spectators a strange groan greeted the verdict, half shock, half dismay. The jury had chosen to disbelieve Marjorie Farber's story. Before the trial she had been warned by Judge Simmill that her testimony might render her liable to prosecution. She acknowledged the risk but said that she wanted to testify anyway. In the event, so complete was the rout of the prosecution's case against Coppolino that the State of New Jersey declined to proceed against her. Unless Marjorie Farber chose to incriminate herself again, there wasn't a hope of proving that a murder had taken place.

Round one had clearly gone to Carl Coppolino.

• • •

The next day, still in custody, Coppolino flew down to Tampa, Florida. During the flight he appeared relaxed and confident, joking with reporters. His head was full of grandiose schemes. Drink in hand, he talked of writing a syndicated newspaper column on medicine and public health. "I'll have to get a public relations man," he bragged. "You know as well as I do that every damned TV show and radio program is going to be after me."

He left behind him a jubilant defense team. They had won the tough trial. Bailey announced to the press that he now expected Florida to withdraw the charge pending against Coppolino. His optimism proved groundless. When Florida reaffirmed its intention of proceeding, Bailey petulantly demanded a change of venue. He didn't want to tackle any redneck Sarasota jury; far better to take his chances in a big city like Miami. Bailey received his change of venue all right—Naples, a sleepy Gulf Coast town with attitudes so deeply entrenched in the nineteenth century that most of its inhabitants viewed Sarasota as a modern-day likeness of Sodom and Gomorrah. Glumly, the defense team prepared itself for the worst.

This time the prosecution left nothing in the bag. They opened their case before Justice Lynn Silvertooth in early April 1967 and State Attorney Frank Schaub had done his homework well. He was a tenacious prosecutor with a fine record. Eighty-five times Schaub had fought capital cases and had won convictions in eighty-two. This was the biggest case of his career, and he was in no mood to lose it.

Recognizing that there was no direct evidence to link Carl Coppolino with the death of his wife, Schaub stacked up a mountain of inconsistencies and a motive for murder that the defense could not answer. High on the list was money. Schaub leaned heavily on the fact that Coppolino had been running short of cash. A couple real estate deals had gone sour and he no longer had Carmela's income to support him. Combine that with the very real possibility that his insurance benefit might be suspended at any time, and it wasn't hard to paint a picture of a desperate man at the end of his financial tether.

Schaub piled it on, characterizing Coppolino as a heartless philanderer, hell-bent on marrying Mary Gibson for her sizable fortune. But Carmela's refusal to grant him a divorce blew that idea sky-high. Instead, Coppolino began eyeing the insurance money, all $65,000. With that, and Mary's bank account, he would be set up for life. There's your motive, Schaub told the jury; could anything be clearer?

Persuasive as Schaub's case was, other, perhaps more significant, forces were at work on his behalf. There persisted in the Naples courtroom an undeniable attitude of "Well, Coppolino might have gotten away with it up north, but he sure as hell ain't gonna make fools of us down here." Nothing was said, of course, but this particular jury gave Milton Helpern a more favorable hearing than its New Jersey counterpart. Helpern's task was much the same as before, to explain the presence of succinylcholine chloride in Carmela's body, and this he did in lucid terms that anyone could understand. The jury also took kindly to toxicology expert Charles Umberger, a former farm boy from Oklahoma with a fondness for chewing tobacco and untidy suits. Before entering the dock, Umberger threw the jury a broad wink. They hung on his every word.

But the final nail in Coppolino's coffin was hammered in by his old nemesis, Marjorie Farber. She testified to overhearing Coppolino on the phone after Carmela's death, saying, "They have started the arterial work and that

won't show anything." Further questioning clarified that
this referred to the fluid used by embalmers to replace the
blood. Marge went on to describe a conversation she had
had with Coppolino just after Carmela's death. In it
Coppolino admitted telling Carmela that their marriage
was over and he wanted a divorce. Carmela had reiterated
her stance that a divorce was out of the question. It was
damning evidence.

Once again Bailey fought like an alley cat but all the
witnesses stood firm. And this time he received no assistance from the defendant. Unaccountably, Coppolino refused to testify on his own behalf. Bailey was stunned,
later calling it "a terrible mistake." The ace defender found
himself in the position of a poker player who has run his
final bluff.

Certainly the jury thought so. After a lengthy deliberation they found Carl Coppolino guilty of second degree
murder, a curious verdict that has never been fully explained since, under Florida law, murder in the second degree indicates a lack of premeditation on the part of the
killer, and anything more premeditated than willful poisoning is hard to imagine. Whatever the reasoning, their decision saved Coppolino from death row. Instead, ashen
faced, the slender ex-doctor who thought he had carried
out the perfect murder was led from the court to begin a
life sentence at Raiford State Prison.

The two Coppolino trials are fascinating for several reasons, but primarily for the insight they give us into the
workings of a jury's mind. In New Jersey the jury was presented with direct evidence from someone who claimed to
have participated in murder. They heard a woman risk the
electric chair in order to tell her story. A more vivid expo-
sition of guilt is hard to imagine. But they chose to acquit.

In Florida, where the evidence was purely circumstantial—and pretty skimpy at that—the jury brought in a verdict of guilty. Had the order of the trials been reversed, it is highly likely that Coppolino would have walked, a free man, from the courthouse. That he did not is due almost entirely to the notoriety attached to his name.

These contrasting trials also highlight the attention that juries pay to the human element when weighing their decision. To see a defiant witness slowly crumble beneath a devastating cross-examination and then slink from the witness box is powerfully compelling. Arcane facts and forensic opinions assailed in a similar fashion have a habit of holding up much better. Most of us are prepared to believe the worst of any person, but we just can't bring ourselves to find fault with a juicy set of incriminating circumstances.

After the second trial, Bailey went on the TV talk-show circuit, campaigning against the verdict's absurdity. His criticism of the Florida legal system went a long way to ensuring that Coppolino's appeals withered on the vine and, ultimately, lawyer and client had an acrimonious parting of the ways.

Carl Coppolino served twelve and a half years of his life sentence until gaining parole in 1979. Prison life obviously proved beneficial as it brought about a miraculous reversal of the heart ailment that had so disabled him two decades earlier. Defying all known medical precedent, Coppolino's much discussed heart condition actually improved with age. On his release he moved back to the Tampa area to be with his wife, Mary. Shortly thereafter he published an account of his years in jail. He called the book *The Crime That Never Was*. Not surprisingly, rancour was evident on every page.

So were the protestations of innocence.

2. THE BROTHERHOOD OF SILENCE

American doctors learn early, in medical school, the folly of exposing malpractice or ethical neglect among their colleagues. The reason is simple: no one wants to jeopardize a promising career by being branded as a troublemaker. After all, the reasoning goes, next time it might be your name under the microscope. As a consequence, many otherwise honorable physicians willfully overlook practices that they know are wrong, all in the interests of self-preservation.

Hospitals, too, keep a tight lid on any wrongdoing. Doctors guilty of grave misconduct can fear censure and immediate dismissal, but little else. The official blanket of secrecy will, in all probability, protect them. References might be terse but any mention of the offense is omitted. This tight-lipped unwillingness on the part of the medical community to share its knowledge has created a haven for the incompetent and the criminal. There is always another job somewhere. At best this shabby system is a disgrace to America. At worst it can lead to disasters like the shame-

ful and wholly preventable career of Dr. Charles Edward
Friedgood.

Many coworkers were aware of this Brooklyn physician's checkered job history—botched and unnecessary
surgeries, multiple firings from half a dozen hospitals. Still
others knew about his financial shenanigans. Some even
heard the rumors suggesting far worse. But the unwritten
code of silence ensured his survival. Not once did a colleague or hospital ever report him to the American Medical
Association. Friedgood continued to butcher and rob patients with absolute impunity, leading a seemingly
charmed existence. Dubious business deals, accusations of
tax evasion, court trials, love affairs conducted in the full
glare of family and friends, illegitimate children—
Friedgood breezed through them all, unaffected and unconcerned. Each incident merely reinforced his perception
of his own invincibility. Given this track record it was perhaps inevitable that such a man would fancy his chances of
getting away with murder.

He very nearly did . . .

August 5, 1975. British Airways' flight 510 from Kennedy
Airport in New York to London was leaving on time. At 10
PM it taxied away from the terminal gate into a sultry summer night. The big jet was half empty. Grateful passengers
began staking out claims to the vacant seats. The more
conscientious among them heeded the attendants' preflight
safety routine. But most were readying themselves for the
long transatlantic flight. Four rows from the front, a mid-
dleaged man with crinkly gray hair and hornrimmed spec-
tacles sat expressionless. Every so often he glanced down
at the black bag lying between his legs, as if reassuring
himself that it was still there. Then he would give another
nervous glimpse through the window at the fading termi-

nal lights. Not long now. In London he would transfer to another plane, this time bound for Denmark, where his mistress and their two children awaited him.

Just another few hours.

Flight 510 gathered speed, rumbling out toward the main runway. Behind it a scene was evolving that might have come straight from the last reel of a Hollywood movie.

Amid a clamor of sirens and flashing lights, the police patrol car swerved and slewed in through the airport gate, then raced across the tarmac. Inside, two detectives scanned the airfield. One of them pointed. Directly ahead they could see the big British Airways jet. Gut feeling told them that this was the one. Had to be. But they were too late. Helplessly they watched the plane slot into the take-off rotation. Frustration ran their nerves ragged. Both cops felt like punching big holes in the dashboard. The person they had come to arrest was about to disappear before their eyes.

In one last-ditch effort, they raised Port Authority HQ on the car radio. Officers there immediately contacted the air traffic control tower. The message was straightforward and uncompromising. "Get ahold of flight 510. There is a murder suspect on board."

At the far end of the airfield the cumbersome jet lumbered awkwardly through 90 degrees onto the main runway. Attendants bustled through the aisles, checking that everyone was safely strapped in. The bespectacled passenger gave one last look out of the window. Far off, the megawatt brightness of Manhattan lit up the nighttime sky. He wondered if he would ever see it again. In his pocket was a ticket for British Airways' earlier flight at eight o'clock, the one he had meant to catch but missed. The delay could have cost him dearly. Still, no problem. He was in the clear now. Sighing, he sank back in his seat and listened to the sweet music of the engines as they howled in readiness for takeoff.

The detectives watched from gate two, unable to believe their eyes. Instead of bolting down the runway, flight 510 had meekly turned and headed back toward them at the terminal.

They had him!

A British Airways security officer came up, demanding to know what was going on. They told him. He went off and returned with details of the seating arrangements. Together, all three men boarded the plane.

The bespectacled passenger watched them approach. A sudden furriness turned his mouth to cotton. The three men stopped beside him. In a discreet voice one of the officers asked him for identification. The passenger produced his passport.

After examining it briefly the officer said, "Would you come with me, please?"

"Is this the thing in Nassau?" asked the passenger, as polite as ever.

"Yes, it is."

"All right."

Charles Edward Friedgood stood up. A tall man. Late fifties. Handsome in a rumpled sort of way. The other passengers must have wondered why he merited such attention. Under their curious gaze, Friedgood left the plane in custody. In his hand was the black overnight bag. He seemed reluctant to part with it . . . understandably, as it contained stolen property worth $600,000.

So very close . . .

From the very start, people felt edgy in his company. Classmates at Central High in Detroit recalled blond, good-looking Charles Friedgood as always being different, not quite one of the guys. Despite the glib personality and a nearly permanent smile, they regarded him as sly. At exam time he cheated blatantly. And he didn't give a damn who knew it. Complaints or inquiries all received his unvarying, enigmatic smile. He was indifferent to the norms of everyday life. In years to come, psychiatry would term the response as sociopathic. For the time being Charlie Friedgood's acquaintances had to make do with old-fashioned words like *ruthless* and *aloof*. Others simply described him as a bastard.

In 1940 he began attending medical school at the University of Michigan. All went well until his final year when it became apparent that a previous history of tuberculosis would seriously hamper his future employment prospects. At that time any suggestion of TB was enough to preclude someone from practicing medicine. Friedgood sent out his job applications and saw them all returned. He decided to set the record straight. He stole some stationery from the dean's office and forged a reference for himself, omitting any mention of the illness. But he went too far, touting himself in such glowing terms that one prospective employer contacted the dean to inquire about this remarkable young man. Friedgood was asked to explain himself, came up short and got kicked out of medical school. Just the first of a hatful of similar expulsions he would suffer in his career.

What happened next is something of a mystery. With America fighting on two fronts in the Second World War, any college student failing to graduate was obliged to enter wartime service as a private. Friedgood later claimed to have done so, but army records do not bear him out; they had no record of a Charles Edward Friedgood at all. Less mysterious is the way that Friedgood was able to wrangle himself into Wayne University for his senior year. He simply cranked up his legendary charm. Dean Nelson knew all about Friedgood's peccadilloes at Michigan but chose to overlook them, feeling that the young man had paid his debt and deserved a second chance.

Once his education was back on track, Friedgood cast around for ways to improve his financial lot. Tuition was expensive and he had no independent source of income. A couple of his fellow students came from well-off families and through them he began to get invitations to weekend house parties. At one of these he met Geraldine Davidson. Angular and somewhat rawboned, Geraldine was a long way from being the usual Charlie Friedgood date; she did, however, have the advantage of being born into one of Detroit's wealthiest families. Charlie stalked her like a rabbit. It was a lightning courtship. The couple married in December 1945, a glamorous, champagne-filled affair.

Gone were the days of hitching a ride to school for the impoverished student. Now it was chauffeur-driven limousines and dashing convertibles. Friedgood basked in his newfound affluence. Expensive suits, a new wardrobe for his mother. He was always ready to show off in front of his friends, gloating over his great good fortune. He declared himself set for life. But the marriage soon foundered and received its death knell when, in a quite remarkable display of reckless audacity, Friedgood gatecrashed a family board meeting and blithely announced, "I'm here because I want to know where I fit in."

One of Geraldine's uncles leapt to his feet and snarled, "I'll tell you where you fit in." Seconds later the upstart son-in-law was thrown out of the room. Divorce was inevitable and came in 1947. Friedgood went back to medicine.

He graduated from Wayne, did his internship at the

Detroit Receiving Hospital, and found a job immediately. Not just any job, either. It was typical of Friedgood's uncanny ability to shrug off setbacks that he landed a residency at the University of Pennsylvania, under Isidor Ravdin, one of the nation's top surgeons. After studying for a year, however, the residency was abruptly canceled. Like so much in Friedgood's career, details surrounding this particular incident are shrouded in mystery. No reasons were ever made public. But, as usual, he was able to turn disaster into advantage. He secured a position at Mount Sinai Hospital in New York City, then at the peak of its celebrity.

This was the big time. Mount Sinai had a reputation for brilliance and overblown egos. In this rarefied atmosphere the surgeons sliced up their rivals with the same deftness they employed on their patients. If ever Charles Friedgood was to be exposed and expelled permanently from the medical profession it was here. Ironically, exactly the opposite happened. Trading heavily on his relationship with Ravdin, Friedgood wheedled himself into a position of influence out of all proportion to his experience. He had a way of ingratiating himself with the hospital hierarchy that made fellow doctors shake their heads in amazement. They were at a loss to explain it. Friedgood's success extended to his private life—he married again.

Like her predecessor, Sophie Davidowitz came from a wealthy family. She was pretty and vivacious and completely bowled over by Friedgood's charm. Her role, as she saw it, was to be the traditional Jewish mother. To that end she remained in a state of perpetual pregnancy—six children in as many years. Friends questioned the effect on her health. But Sophie wouldn't have it any other way. It was what her Charlie wanted.

By 1950 they were living in Brooklyn to be near

Maimonides Hospital, Friedgood's latest place of employment. It did not take him long to run afoul of the hospital's ethics and standards. He began by conning other doctors out of their patients. Colleagues soon learned to keep a wary eye on Friedgood, who wasn't above sneaking their patients' medical records and penciling his own name in as attending physician. And then there was the money. Always, there was trouble with the money. Maimonides prided itself on a reputation for free medical attention—most of the patients were indigent—but Friedgood wanted no part of that. He began charging for his services. When the hospital authorities found out they were furious and slapped him with a reprimand. Friedgood made a formal apology but continued charging fees, as if nothing had happened.

His ability to align himself with his superiors made him virtually impregnable, even when whispers of downright criminal behavior began to circulate. The nastiest incident concerned a baby operated on by Friedgood for heart problems. Submitting an under-the-counter bill to the family was bad enough, but worse was to follow. When the baby showed no signs of improvement, the concerned parents decided to obtain a second opinion. They took their child to another surgeon. His examination revealed that Friedgood had not performed any surgery at all; he had just made an incision that required suturing.

News of the outrage filtered back to Maimonides and an investigation was set in motion. Although several staff members were aware of Friedgood's appalling misconduct, none felt the need to report him. They later claimed that responsibility lay with their superiors. Passing the buck in order to make a buck, it seemed, was more important than drumming a potentially lethal doctor out of business. Still smiling, Charlie Friedgood continued to practice.

But his days at Maimonides were numbered. A new head of surgery, Alfred Hurwitz, took over. For once, Friedgood's charm failed him. Hurwitz could see right through this slipshod physician with a penchant for stealing patients. After a blazing row, Friedgood was fired. Decades later Hurwitz said he was unable to recall the reason for the row, only the vehemence of Friedgood's threat as he stormed from the office: "I'll kill you . . . If it's the last thing I ever do . . . I'll kill you."

Anxious to avoid any hint of scandal, Maimonides Hospital kept their reservations about Charles Friedgood under wraps. Never again, though, would he work at such a prestigious hospital.

The downward spiral began. In quick succession, Friedgood got himself fired from three lower-echelon hospitals. Even at this level the hospital boards were clannish and reluctant to divulge their reasons, with the result that Friedgood always managed to keep working. By 1960, however, faced by an ever-dwindling job market, he was forced to take a position at lowly Interboro Hospital in Brooklyn. He joined as a partner, the hospital being run by doctors on a consortium basis.

Friedgood's part of the operation was ramshackle, to say the least. His office became a meeting place for the local Hassidim, devoutly orthodox Jews who took Friedgood to their hearts. He became an almost supernatural figure to these people who knew more of the scriptures than they did of life. To them the doctor who treated their illnesses and never charged a penny was inspirational. Little did they know that philanthropic Charlie Friedgood was submitting insurance claims on their behalf to

Medicare and Medicaid. He always found a way to get paid.

Something else that paid well were abortions. No one knows exactly when Friedgood first added this profitable sideline, but by 1964 he was charging up to $1,000 for the then illegal procedure. Even here his clumsiness caught up with him. One of his patients, Evelyn Handelman, had to be rushed, hemorrhaging, to a hospital emergency room. The admitting physician immediately diagnosed an almost fatal abortion. The police were contacted. They garnered enough evidence on Friedgood to warrant tapping his office telephone. Months of surveillance led to eight indictments against Friedgood on charges of performing abortions.

The prosecution put together a cast-iron case, then had the rug yanked from beneath them—Evelyn Handelman refused to testify. Since the abortion, she had married, and her husband, knowing nothing of her trauma, was under the impression that she was *virgo intacta* on their wedding night. Evelyn said that if he was now to learn otherwise, it would destroy the marriage and she would kill herself. There was something in the implacable manner that she imparted this information that made the DA's office sit up and listen. This was no idle threat. Prosecutors put their heads together. Believing they had enough to obtain a conviction on the other seven counts, it was decided to leave the poor woman in peace.

But they had reckoned without Charles Friedgood. He hired a firm of New York lawyers which specialized in tapping cases. They came up with the goods. In March 1965, the State Supreme Court ruled that any evidence obtained by tapping was inadmissible. The prosecution was sunk. Without Evelyn Handelman they didn't have a prayer. Charles Friedgood was able to walk from the courtroom a free man, his reputation virtually intact. He didn't even have to worry about embarrassing media coverage; the case had attracted hardly any local attention.

But if everything was holding together on the professional front, at home it was an entirely different story. In 1959, Sophie, still only thirty-three years old, had suffered a stroke. Her personality changed overnight. Gone was the radiant fun-loving girl that Friedgood had married; in her place was a shrewish, complaining woman, riddled with paranoia and gloom. The couple argued incessantly. Gradually the children began to side with their father in this war. They heard him threaten their mother but put it down to provocation. They understood why he took to staying late at the hospital, even if at times they knew he was with other women. They tolerated all of this because he was their father and they loved him. Ironically, it was the testimony of his own children that finally eclipsed Charles Friedgood. But all of that was several years in the future. For now he had their trust and he had their sympathy.

With his domestic life in tatters, Friedgood began noticing a nurse who worked at Interboro Hospital. Harriet Larsen was from Denmark, no raving beauty but quite handsome and a model of Scandinavian efficiency. She took over the day-to-day running of Friedgood's chaotic office. First of all she straightened out the paperwork, then she went to work on Friedgood, insisting that he tidy up his disheveled appearance. For the first time in his life, Friedgood began getting regular haircuts. He also began taking Harriet to his bed.

His children noticed the change in him and soon learned of his relationship with Harriet. In no time at all Friedgood had everyone on the best of terms. But his recklessness backfired on him badly when he showed up at a graduation party for daughter Debbie with Harriet on his arm. When Sophie saw the two of them together she became hysterical, hurling a shoe at the ice-cool Dane and screaming all manner of insults. Family members had to drag her away. Friedgood merely smiled and carried on as though nothing was happening. This embarrassing incident further alienated the children from their mother. Debbie even went so far as to write complimentary poems to Harriet, privately wishing that she and her father would marry.

In 1971, Harriet became pregnant. At first she claimed that a previous boyfriend was the father, but no one was fooled. She returned to Denmark and there gave birth to a baby boy who was the image of Charles Friedgood. When baby Heinrich—named after Friedgood's father—was three months old, mother and son returned to the States. The relationship between Friedgood and Harriet now took on a more serious air. They openly paraded their son at Interboro Hospital. Friedgood's mother even acted as babysitter while doctor and nurse made their rounds.

But the sands were beginning to shift beneath Friedgood's feet.

Following his 1964 manslaughter trial, he became the subject of intense IRS scrutiny. Government tax collectors wanted to know more about this doctor and his alleged $1,000 abortions. Their investigation took years but they eventually amassed enough evidence for indictment. The trial came to court in the autumn of 1972. The government claimed that Friedgood owed them $400,000 in back taxes and penalties.

Adopting an air of injured innocence, Friedgood said his tax returns had always been completed by his late father. Any errors which might have occurred were entirely the old man's fault. As a plea it had a tired ring to it— blaming a dead man was one of the oldest and most feeble defenses around—and this time Friedgood was found guilty. His tearful protestations of remorse to the court did ensure a lenient sentence—five years probation, payment of all taxes due and a month at a public health facility in Texas. Friedgood promptly began putting all his assets in his wife's name. Contrition, apparently, didn't include any intention of paying the money due.

Some indication of Friedgood's state of mind at this point is evidenced by the fact that, while on trial for tax evasion, he was also the subject of yet another, quite different, grand jury investigation. This time the charge was attempted murder.

The case had its beginnings in 1964 when Friedgood met a businessman named Toby Miller. Miller had recently acquired a Holiday Inn, built on land near JFK airport, for $1.6 million. With the building still incomplete, Miller found himself overextended financially. He needed immediate cash to stave off foreclosure. A mutual friend, Jerry Gottlieb, introduced him to Friedgood. The doctor inspected the half-built hotel and liked what he saw. Using Sophie's money he agreed to buy a 45 percent stake in the venture for $450,000. So desperate was Miller at this point that, when the smiling doctor blithely demanded a $12,500 finder's fee for Gottlieb as a condition of acceptance, he accepted. Making it worse was Friedgood's insistence that the check be made out to his own father. Miller, in no position to argue, gritted his teeth and reached for his checkbook.

Despite this rather undistinguished beginning, the two men became fast friends. The hotel prospered, they met socially, Miller even used to visit Friedgood at the hospital. But gradually their camaraderie waned, in large part because Friedgood felt that Miller was cheating him. To iron out their differences, in 1970 they drew up a complicated buy-sell agreement over their shares in the Holiday Inn. In its simplest form it meant that either party could buy out the other for a fixed sum. Should the seller not be satisfied with the offer, he then had the option to counter within thirty days at a figure 10 percent higher. Another clause, buried deep in the small print and legal jargon, stated that if either party defaulted as purchaser, then the seller could purchase his partner's interest at his original price. Miller, a much shrewder businessman than Friedgood, decided that herein lay the road to independence.

In 1972 he offered $400,000 for Friedgood's share. As the property was now worth at least $2 million, Friedgood immediately countered with 10 percent more. Miller accepted. But Friedgood, as Miller had thought, couldn't come up with anything like that sort of cash. Miller cried foul and said that under the terms of the agreement his original offer of $400,000 was valid and that Friedgood was legally bound to accept. Friedgood became apoplectic. He contacted Miller urgently, requesting a meeting. Miller refused to take his call. Friedgood decided that a personal visit might help things along.

The morning of July 2, 1972, began in the usual way for Toby Miller, according to his subsequent testimony before the grand jury. He left his house at 8 AM, steered his Mercedes down the driveway and onto the quiet dirt road that led to the main highway. Some way along the track a Cadillac barred his path. It appeared to have broken down. Miller drew to a halt and rolled down his window. A heavily built young man got out of the Cadillac and walked over. Before Miller could say a word the stranger had wrenched open the Mercedes door, hurled Miller across the seat and jumped in beside him. A second man ran across from the Cadillac. He stuck his head in through the window and growled something about Miller's dispute with Charles Friedgood. Before Miller could respond a third car drew up. Out of the blue Mustang stepped Charles Friedgood. In his hand was a brown envelope. He hurried over to the Mercedes and climbed in. Miller was now sandwiched between the two men. Friedgood smiled. "I have some papers for you."

He nodded to the young thug who started up the car and drove off. It wasn't far to a deserted lane. They parked. Friedgood ordered Miller to remove his jacket. Miller did as he was told and waited, quaking, as Friedgood calmly filled a syringe.

"Raise your right arm," said Friedgood, injecting Miller below the right armpit. From the envelope Friedgood then produced a stack of legal forms. "Sign these."

"What are they?" gasped Miller.

At this one of the other men snapped, "Don't read 'em. Just sign your name, if you know what's good for you."

With the injection acting fast, Miller signed everything. Ten . . . twelve . . . fifteen . . . he didn't know how many. The last thing he remembered was begging Friedgood to drive him home. Then everything went black.

He came to in his living room. He was alone. Still reeling, he drifted back into unconsciousness. The next time he awoke it was because Charles Friedgood was beating the living daylights out of him, screaming, "I'm going to kill you."

Somehow Miller fought Friedgood off. What he did next was even more remarkable. He convinced the manic Friedgood that they should call an attorney and settle this amicably. Friedgood panted agreement. Miller dialed his lawyer. "Come to my house, quick," he gasped. "Charlie Friedgood tried to kill me!"

Forty minutes later, when the lawyer arrived, Friedgood

was nowhere to be seen. Toby Miller was clearly in a bad way. The lawyer rushed him to the hospital. The attending doctor made a note of the puncture wound under Miller's arm. Also recorded was a barbiturate level in Miller's blood of 4.7 mg, an almost lethal amount. Miller spent four days in intensive care, then another three under observation. As soon as he left the hospital he filed a complaint. Friedgood was arrested and charged with assault, robbery and kidnapping.

The case went before a grand jury. They studied all the evidence and concluded that it was just too fantastic a story to be true. Without a corroborating witness, all they had to go on was Miller's word alone. It wasn't enough. The case was dismissed. Charlie Friedgood's lucky charm had worked again.

Soon afterward he got into more trouble, this time at Interboro Hospital. The complaint centered on a notorious fault of his, unpunctuality. He had kept a patient waiting in the operating theater. The anesthesiologist, assuming that Friedgood would arrive at any moment, continued sedating the child. But something went sadly wrong. The child died. Blame for the tragedy was laid squarely at Friedgood's door. The hospital decided that they had finally had enough of Charles Friedgood and gave him his marching orders.

He began a slow descent, working fly-by-night Brooklyn clinics. But he couldn't escape his problems. He got nailed with a malpractice suit, and this time not even Charlie Friedgood's legendary luck could pull him through.

One of his patients, Nanette Edelstein, unhappy about the size of her breasts, decided to try plastic surgery to enlarge them. Friedgood performed a routine breast-implant operation, even though he had no history of cosmetic surgery. His shortcomings were soon evident. The restructured breasts assumed a strange shape and began oozing an unpleasant pus. Four times Friedgood tried to remedy the mess he had made of the operation but the problem continued to worsen. Eventually the poor woman went to another physician. What she learned horrified her—Dr. Charles Friedgood had inserted the breast implants upside down. She filed a complaint.

Lack of insurance coverage—his underwriters declined liability because he was operating outside his field of expertise—left Friedgood without the money to afford an attorney. For someone of his sensibilities it was a minor inconvenience. He defended himself. After a few rough spots, such as hurling a briefcase at opposing counsel and storming petulantly from the court, Friedgood did a very competent job. It was enough to earn the respect of his trial adversaries but not of the jury. They decided in Nanette Edelstein's favor, awarding $65,000 damages. Even so, Friedgood got off lightly. Press coverage of the trial was minimal and no professional body saw fit to conduct an investigation into this doctor with the appalling record. His license remained intact.

And he still had Harriet. If anything the relationship grew stronger, especially when, in 1974, Harriet became pregnant again. As before, she returned to Denmark for the birth. This time Friedgood joined her there and they flew back to the States together. But now Harriet became more demanding, insisting that Friedgood leave his wife. Friedgood explained that, because of the litigation with Miller, all his money was tied up in Sophie's name; separation was impossible. Disenchanted, Harriet booked a flight back to Denmark.

When Sophie learned of Harriet's departure, she underwent a remarkable transformation. Real hope came back into her life. She lost weight and generally smartened up her appearance. She also told the children that there hadn't really been anything to the affair at all. The children, kindly, said nothing. Even when Sophie found a batch of letters and a photograph of Harriet's first baby, she chose to pretend nothing had happened. It was all very sad. The tragedy of Sophie Friedgood was that she genuinely loved her husband, always had and always would. The thought of life without him was totally abhorrent to her. She would rather die than lose Charlie. Unfortunately, her husband was of the same mind.

The world must have looked good to Sophie Friedgood on June 17, 1975: no mistress to worry about and every reason to believe that things between her and Charlie were on the mend. On that afternoon she and a partner reached the final of their golf club tournament. Sophie celebrated by buying a couple of golf bags in the pro shop, one for herself and one for Charlie. Later that evening she had a dinner engagement with her husband at a local restaurant. As always, Charlie was late, but the dinner passed pleasantly enough and, after stopping off to see their accountant, the couple went home to their rambling Long Island house. A friend telephoned and spoke to them both. They seemed in good spirits. Sometime around eleven o'clock they got ready for bed.

What happened next can only be guessed at. As the prosecution later told it, Friedgood went to a cabinet in his study and there filled a hypodermic syringe with Demerol, a powerful painkiller. Then he retraced his steps to the bedroom. Sophie lay naked on the bed. Friedgood approached, smiling. In an instant he grabbed hold of Sophie's arms, yanked them upwards and rammed the needle deep into her side. Demerol is not especially fast acting, so it is probable that Friedgood had to hold his wife facedown on the bed to smother her screams. A few minutes later, when

Sophie lapsed into delirium, he injected her several more times, culminating in a shot straight into the liver. Her eyes fell shut.

Friedgood returned the syringe to the study cabinet. A short while later he came back across the hallway to the bedroom. Sophie was dead. Friedgood obviously found all this exertion quite fatiguing, because his final action of the night was to crawl into bed beside his dead wife and fall fast asleep.

The next day the body of Sophie Friedgood lay undiscovered till after lunch. A friend phoned and was alarmed to hear from the maid, Lydia, that Sophie was still in bed. Better check on her, she said. The maid tried to rouse Sophie from what she thought was a deep sleep. Then she noticed the cold, blue lips. She ran back to the phone and blurted out, "Mrs. Friedgood no waking up." The friend immediately dialed 911.

When Friedgood got the message, he rushed home. The police and paramedics were already there. Friedgood ran upstairs to the bedroom. Faced by the sight of Sophie's plump naked body, he broke down. He began kissing her, sobbing, "My Sophie, my Sophie, she's dead." A policeman comforted him. In between the tears Friedgood told how his wife had a history of strokes; he'd been half-expecting something like this.

Then Friedgood did a most peculiar thing. He signed the death certificate himself, listing the cause as a "cerebral vascular accident" or stroke. At that time in New York State, there was no law against a doctor signing another family member's death certificate, but it was unofficially frowned upon. To do so was bound to attract suspicion. Friedgood had made his first blunder.

His second came shortly afterward when he announced that, in accordance with orthodox Jewish law, Sophie had to be interred before sundown the following day. There was an eagerness to his manner that police found disquieting. Soon they began thinking that all was not well with Dr. Charles Edward Friedgood.

Sophie's body was shipped to her family in Hazleton, Pennsylvania, for burial. Back at the Nassau County Police Department an argument was raging over whether to pull Friedgood in. Finally it was decided to confront him. Three officials drove down to Hazleton. They caught up with Friedgood at the funeral director's office and bluffed him into agreeing to an autopsy. Friedgood did have one proviso. He insisted on being present. The police were not empowered to deny his request but could not recall another instance of a grieving husband requesting to be present while the body of his wife was carved up for forensic inspection. It only served to intensify their suspicions.

During the autopsy several damaging anomalies came to light. First, the stomach was very full. As food generally evacuates the stomach within six hours, it was clear that Sophie Friedgood died soon after eating a large meal. Since it was known that she had not eaten breakfast, death must have occurred after the previous night's dinner. This did not square with Friedgood's assertion that his wife had been fine when he had left for work that morning. It was not medically possible.

There was also the motif of yellow-and-black bruises, caused by the hypodermic needle. Friedgood said they were inflicted after death. The doctor who performed the autopsy thought otherwise. He ordered samples from the body to be sent for forensic analysis. The toxicologist had no trouble establishing the presence of 600 mg of Demerol, more than twice a fatal dose. The only difficulty he had was in believing that a fellow physician could be stupid enough to use such an easily detected drug.

Police lost no time in obtaining a warrant to search Friedgood's house. They arrived in the middle of deep family mourning. Relatives were coming and going nonstop. Friedgood greeted the official intrusion glumly but did not attempt to stop it. The search began. When the chaos was at its peak he drew one of his daughters, Esther, into a corner and whispered, first in Yiddish, then English, "Upstairs. File cabinet. Bottle. Syringe. Top drawer."

Frightened and confused, Esther crept to the study where she found the bottle and syringe. At a loss for what to do, she stuffed them into a paper bag, then hid the package in her underwear. After the police finished searching one of the bedrooms, she hid the parcel there. The only person she told was her father. Three days later, when Esther went to check on the parcel, it was gone.

Friedgood realized the game was up. He began a frantic round of safe-deposit boxes and bank vaults, looting his wife's estate of both jewelery and bonds. Then he made his last and biggest mistake. While at the airport he called his family to say that he was going away for a few days; heart trouble, he said. Because of all the background noise, someone asked Friedgood if he was at the airport. Friedgood hedged. The hesitation finished him. His son-in-law, Abraham Meneshe, already suspicious about Sophie's death, contacted the police. Minutes later the chase to JFK airport began.

Charles Friedgood was convicted by his own children. Their testimony stripped him bare. Esther told the court about the Demerol and the syringe. The others recounted his mistreatment of their mother. Friedgood had no defense at all. On December 15, 1976, he was found guilty of murder. A month later he was back in court for sentencing. Looking haggard and drawn, he made an impassioned plea on his own behalf: "I know I am innocent, and I have to be put away for the rest of my life. This isn't justice . . . I swear to you, Judge, I did not commit this crime."

Judge Richard C. Delin was not impressed. He told Friedgood, "You were motivated by greed and lust—greed for your wife's jewels and lust for your mistress. You utilized your skill as a physician to administer five doses of Demerol . . . This was no crime of passion. You persisted until your goal was accomplished." The judge then passed the maximum sentence, twenty-five years to life imprisonment.

Charlie Friedgood's luck had finally run out.

Some good came of this disaster. In 1978 the New York State Legislature passed a law prohibiting doctors from signing any death certificate for a relative. The tall, gray-haired inmate serving time at the Fishkill Correction Facility in Beacon would have been furious to learn that legislators referred to the bill as the "Friedgood Law."

3. THE MARRYING KIND

Multiple murderers, like most other career criminals, are creatures of habit. They find a method that works and stick with it. For this streak of conservatism, the general public should be grateful. Enough repetition invariably leads to arrest. After all, it wasn't any great feat of criminal detection that brought George Joseph Smith, the "Brides in the Bath" murderer to the gallows, but rather a lynx-eyed newspaper reader who noticed that the latest of Smith's wives had died in remarkably similar circumstances to those of her predecessor and informed the police.

So it was with Dr. Robert George Clements. For most of his adult life this bluff and burly Irishman had acquired and dispatched wives with no great fuss or suspicion. True, each bereavement coincided with a precipitous drop in the wife's finances, but a fondness for travel and the limited communications of the day spared Clements any embarrassing brushes with the law. Had he kept on the move it is possible that Clements could have avoided detection altogether. But in his dotage the doctor became slipshod. More than that, he became foolish. Maybe it was the brisk Southport air in the northwest of England, rushing in off the Irish Sea, that turned his silvery head; maybe the first knockings of senility. Whatever the reason, in 1947 Dr. Clements did something downright stupid—he went to the murderer's well just once too often.

There was nothing in his background to indicate the mayhem to come. The Clements family was well respected in Dungannon, a small town in County Tyrone, Ireland. Good Protestant stock, comfortably set financially, able to send all four sons to college. After graduation, Robert, the youngest, followed his eldest brother into medicine (the remaining two brothers chose those other stalwart professions of the Victorian middle class, the ministry and the armed services). Both at school and afterward, Clements made a name for himself on the sporting field. His husky build and competitiveness made him a natural athlete. He had talent, as well, enough to represent his country at both lacrosse and rugby. In the classroom he was equally successful. His MB came in 1904. Four years later, at the age of twenty-eight, he qualified as a doctor in Belfast.

Even in college he demonstrated a zest for the more exotic things in life—sumptuous meals, the theater, nightclubs and women, always women. They were drawn hypnotically to him. It was hardly surprising. Robert Clements's line of Irish blarney could charm the pigeons out of the sky. Tack on to that his celebrity as a sportsman and those undeniable good looks and the young man from Dungannon had it made. Except for one thing—money.

As an impecunious young general practitioner struggling to make his way in the world, he was constantly short of money. In no way could he sustain the lifestyle he craved without a radical improvement in his financial situation. Something would have to be done. His solution? Supremely simple: marry someone with the means and temperament to sponsor his chosen way of life.

He had to wait until 1912. It proved to be a bumper year all round. Not only did Clements finally catch that wife he'd been after, but he was also admitted as a Fellow of the Royal College of Surgeons, Edinburgh. There is little doubt which triumph accorded him the most satisfaction. Earning the respect of one's peers might do wonders for the ego, but couldn't begin to compare with the pecuniary benefits of landing an heiress.

It speaks volumes for the homeliness of Edyth Mercier's nature and appearance that, despite being the daughter of one of Belfast's wealthiest corn merchants, she had been able to reach early middle age without tripping up the aisle. Ever the pragmatist, Clements was fully prepared to overlook Edyth's physical shortcomings and the ten-year gap in their ages and instead concentrate on the really important side of their relationship—her bank balance. He was aided marvelously in this respect by the bride's father who, possibly relieved to have rid himself of a forty-two-year-old and exceedingly plain daughter, settled a very large sum of money on the couple at the time of their marriage.

Clements had hit the jackpot. And things kept getting better. Just eighteen months later Mr. Mercier, by now a patient of his son-in-law, succumbed to cancer. For the first time Clements signed one of those death certificates that were to play such an important and beneficial role in his life. When the old man's will was proven, it showed that he had settled another £25,000 on his daughter, worth well over a quarter of a million in present-day terms.

Not surprising, Robert and Edyth Clements were popular in Belfast society. They occupied a large detached house in one of the city's more prestigious areas, joined all the fashionable local associations and entertained on a lavish scale. Neither did Clements cut back on his amorous ramblings. Shrugging off the encumbrance of a wife, Clements bulldozed into one affair after another with a brazenness that became the talk of Belfast. Like so many medical men who have resorted to murder, Clements had unlimited reserves of vanity. In his eyes, the social prestige of his calling seemed to preclude any possibiity that he would be held accountable for his actions. He trampled conventional social mores underfoot, a law unto himself.

In time, of course, the gossip reached Edyth's ears. To general surprise, she did nothing. It's conceivable that she did not believe the stories, but far more probable is the likelihood that she chose to ignore them altogether. If nothing else Edyth was a realist. In those days unattractive divorcées did not rate very highly on the social scale. If she wanted to remain married, she had little choice but to overlook her husband's blatant infidelities. Besides, there was another reason. By 1920 Edyth desperately needed the security of marriage. She was broke, down to her last few pounds. In just eight years Dr. Robert Clements had cleaned out the joint account and blown the lot.

When Edyth found out, she complained bitterly to Clements, but he swept her grievances aside with his usual blend of charm and guile. "Nothing to worry about," he coaxed. "Anyway, Edyth, someone in your condition shouldn't go working themselves up over nothing."

Edyth had to admit he was right. For some months, now, she had been feeling unwell, tired all the time, often too weak to stand. Yes, she really should take things more easily. But it didn't do any good. Her condition worsened. "Sleeping sickness," Clements sighed to concerned friends, a tropical disease notorious for its low survival rate. He added somberly that it was "only a matter of time." His warning proved uncannily prophetic. Within days of the prediction, in the autumn of 1920, Edyth died. Clements, barely able to control his grief, somehow mustered the wherewithal to sign the death certificate himself.

With the funeral over, he became itchy. Belfast was too small, too provincial and definitely too dangerous for what he had in mind. Like so many of his countrymen before him, Clements began eyeing the opportunities that existed just across the Irish Sea. England, that was the place. A man could make his way in England. No shortage of available women either, the Great War had seen to that. Suitably primed, Clements sold his Belfast practice and packed his bags, off in search of another well-to-do spouse.

He settled in Manchester. Maybe the glory days were gone, but there was still enough money gushing through the city that liked to term itself "The Capital of the North" to keep the speculators happy. Fortunes made in cotton were flaunted in the private clubs, and there came face to face with the peripatetic Dr. Clements. He had a ready smile and a sympathetic ear and, before long, began picking up invitations to house parties—eligible men were an endangered species in postwar Manchester—that brought him a solid circle of patients. Clements never missed a trick. Becoming a Freemason didn't hurt. Neither did his charm. He still had it in spades. Women were attracted to him in droves. Most were pretty, all were rich.

From out of the pack Mary McCreary emerged as the likeliest contender for matrimony. She was the daughter of a wealthy Manchester industrial magnate whose family also hailed from Ireland. Clements, trading heavily on his Gaelic background, won her over in record time. Less than a year after Edyth's death, in the summer of 1921,

Clements led his new bride down the aisle, no doubt pondering how he could spend the very sizeable sum of money that Mary's father had donated by way of a wedding gift.

Back in the financial saddle again, Clements stepped up his social activity. This time, however, he had to severely curtail his extramarital dalliances. Mary was not the pushover that Edyth had been and kept him on a much tighter rein. It may not have been entirely coincidental that Clements chose this moment to start a family. With the arrival of son George in 1923, Mary's ability to act as watchdog suffered a crippling setback. She was a virtual prisoner in her own home, powerless to learn what her husband was up to. This was probably just as well because Clements was acting the goat again. He was also spending her money at a staggering rate.

Coincidentally, as the money dwindled so did Mary's health until, by 1925, there was very little left of either. Clements put the word around that Mary was suffering from a heart condition—"Serious," said the doctor. He laid the groundwork well. When Mary expired, no one expressed any great astonishment. The death certificate, again furnished by a sorrowful Clements, recorded the cause as "endocarditis." Everyone agreed it was a tragedy.

Soon afterward, Clements took a break from his role of professional husband, dumped son George on some relatives, and went to sea as a ship's doctor. For much of the next two years he steamed around the Orient. A veil of mystery hangs over this time abroad. Clements did not show his face again until 1927 when he reappeared in Manchester. Just about the only visible evidence of his Oriental sojourn was the Japanese manservant he brought back with him. Such an aberration in staid Manchester raised more than one eyebrow but proved to be a useful talking point as Clements reestablished his practice and set about proving himself once again as a social lion.

He'd lost none of his charisma. An endless stream of wealthy socialites beat a path to his ever-open door. He wined, dined and bedded them all with equal gusto. Quite a contest was developing to see who would be the third Mrs. Clements when the medical Don Juan pulled a stroke that floored most of the competition. In 1928 he abruptly married longtime family friend Kathleen Burke. Not only had she personally known both of her predecessors, but Kathleen also had the singular distinction—at least as far as Clements was concerned—of hardly having any money at all. In the absence of any evidence to the contrary, one can only assume that this time Clements married with the best of intentions. If so, it was his one brush with decency.

With the money he had saved abroad and his income from a successful practice, Clements was just about able to sustain himself in the lifestyle to which he had become accustomed. True, he couldn't be quite so extravagant as before, but any cutbacks he made were so marginal as to be hardly noticeable. To further bolster funds, he began dabbling in esoteric forms of medicine. Viewed from this distance of time, much of what he prescribed smacks of quackery, but in the early thirties there were many who swore by the benefits of hydrotherapy, a form of water cure. Another, somewhat more drastic, form of treatment that Clements employed was the administration of medicine by means of suppositories and anal douches. Unattractive work, but it paid the bills.

In 1933 Clements, by then well into his fifties, opted for semiretirement. He and Kathleen moved south and took over the running of a hotel in the New Forest. It was an ill-starred venture. With the Depression hitting hard, there was little spare cash around for hotel rooms and Clements was forced to take on temp work to make ends meet. His frequent absences meant that Kathleen had to run the hotel virtually on her own. Her health, never robust at the best of times, rebelled under the strain. Exacerbating the problem was her instinctive dislike of living in the south. She was a northern girl, born and bred, unable to get along with people she considered rude and standoffish. Because of this, in 1935 they sold the hotel and moved back north, this time to the Lancashire seaside town of Southport.

If Clements intended resuming his practice, then he could not have chosen a more suitable venue. Southport was, and to some extent still is, a town favored by the elderly for their retirement years. They come for the bracing winds and unhurried ways and to be among their own kind. For many the trip is a short one, just eighteen miles up the road from the swaggering sprawl and brawl of Liverpool. A brief journey, maybe, but Southport, with its air of faded gentility, discreet money and an invincible upper-middle class, is light years removed from its neighbor to the south.

Clements knew this. There would be no shortage of patients and, given the above average number of wealthy widows, no dearth of romantic interest, either. He and Kathleen settled in quickly. Many of their old friends from Manchester often made the trip over to see them. Soon it was the familiar swirl of restaurants and theaters, parties and nightclubs. A casual observer might have been excused for thinking that Clements was ideally set, but beneath his facile veneer of contentment the doctor was in turmoil. Not only had the hotel been a disaster financially, but the small amount of capital that Kathleen called her own was now entirely gone—hardly Clements's idea of marital bliss. He began looking for a way out.

Deciding to murder Kathleen must have caused him much soul-searching. On the one hand was the genuine affection he clearly felt for his latest wife, but against this had to be balanced a craving for money that was well nigh insatiable. In 1938 he reluctantly reached his decision. Almost immediately Kathleen's health began to fail and she was taken to the Kenworthy Hydro. On this occasion Clements did not attend his wife but instead called in another practitioner. However, this didn't prevent him from making strong suggestions as to what was ailing Kathleen—tuberculosis—and gloomily forecasting her imminent demise. He got it right almost to the day. At Clements's behest the attending physician duly signed the death certificate, confirming TB as the cause.

Robert Clements cut an impressive figure at the funeral in his mourning black, nearing sixty and fashionably stout, with as much silver in his hair as he had in his tongue. He was dignified and he was tragic, and he was possessed of an apparently foolproof method for getting away with murder.

Or so it seemed.

Only many years later was it learned that the death of his third wife, far from slipping by unnoticed, had come perilously close to unmasking Robert Clements. He had avoided arrest by a hair's breadth.

Irene Gayus, another Southport doctor, had known Kathleen for years, not as a patient but as a very close friend. Blessed with a skeptical nature and unimpressed by affectation, Irene was distrustful of Clements from the beginning. She found his line of glib bonhomie jarring and bogus. Gut instinct told her that Kate had married a wrong 'un. Whether she confided these misgivings to Kathleen is not known, but Irene Gayus does seem to have been something of an amateur detective. Contact with friends in Manchester brought news of Clements's scandalous reputation and his previous wife's sudden demise when her money was gone. Further digging uncovered details of the first Mrs. Clements in Belfast. Irene's curiosity grew into outright suspicion when she found that, on both occasions, Clements himself had signed the death certificate. While not illegal, Irene Gayus, as a physician, was quick to spot the lack of ethics in such a procedure. Nudging the amateur sleuth along in her inquiries was the knowledge that, in the final weeks before Kathleen's death, Clements had been seen openly squiring another, very rich, lady around the shops and salons of Southport.

When Kathleen died, Dr. Gayus could contain herself no longer. She rushed to the chief constable of Southport, Lieutenant-Colonel Harold Mighall, and poured out her story. He listened intently to what she had to say and admitted that it sounded very suspicious. After consulting the coroner, Mighall ordered a postmortem.

Unfortunately, he was just a matter of hours too late. That very morning Kathleen Clements had been cremated in Liverpool. Her husband, according to the other mourners, was positively distraught. So were the authorities; without a body they didn't have a prayer.

If Clements ever heard of, or suspected, this official interest in his activities—and it's hard to believe in gossipy prewar Southport that he didn't—then he certainly did not show it. On the contrary, he plunged straight back into the social swim and, in a matter of months, was eagerly courting Amy Victoria Barnett, twenty years his junior and another lady of means. Once again, Dame Fortune shone on the persistent suitor. Amy's father, a Liverpool industrial tycoon, died unexpectedly in January 1940, leaving her £22,000. To help her over the shock, Clements proposed marriage. Amy, who preferred to be known as "Vee," consented with barely a second thought.

Despite the wartime restrictions, their marriage in London was a spectacular affair. Clements's own brother, William, conducted the ceremony at fashionable St. George's Church in Hanover Square, while son George acted as usher. For the reception, a banquet was laid on at the Mayfair Hotel where several hundred guests gorged themselves on the plentiful array of food. After a short honeymoon "somewhere in the south of England," the happy couple returned to Southport, and the luxury and splendor of an eight-room flat at 20 The Promenade, formerly occupied by Vee's father. From his window, Clements could gaze out across the Irish Sea, glad, perhaps, to put all those memories behind him.

Flush once again, Clements cut down drastically on his private practice and stepped up his socializing. But in 1940, as the so-called "Phony War" gave way to the real thing, and more young doctors were called up for active duty, he found himself seconded to fill the vacuum they left.

He took a post as deputy medical officer of health for Blackburn, daily commuting back and forth from Southport. It was important work but not overly time consuming and afforded him ample opportunity to indulge his two main interests, the local Conservative Party and writing papers for submission to the *Lancet* and the *British Medical Journal*. Throughout the war he and his wife remained prominent in Southport society. Vee, in particular, was very keen on amateur theatricals and the church, and encouraged her husband similarly. Clements proved to be a capable actor but preferred to spend his evenings at the local Masonic lodge, or so he told Vee.

While no one could deny the couple's sociability, they did have one quirk which gave rise to speculation. It concerned their flat on The Promenade. Guests were only admitted into the elegantly furnished drawing room where they could gaze on the impressive grand piano, the display case of Dresden china and some fine oil paintings. The rest of the flat was strictly off limits. Clements was most insistent about this. Any inquiry about what lay behind those closed doors was politely deflected. But beneath the charming smile lay a steely resolution. Only years later would the reason for this become known.

At the end of the war, Clements found himself in virtual retirement. He was now sixty-five years old and the rigors of a full and active life were beginning to show in his leathery face. But the brain was as active as ever, and so were certain other organs. If only he didn't have Vee around . . .

Her sickness began in December of 1946, and took the form of violent headaches, giddiness and loss of memory. Out in the car one day, she collapsed and had to be rushed home. Jaundice, Clements informed friends sadly. Later, he announced that the trouble had spread to her gall bladder and that he was requesting a second opinion.

Dr. John Holmes listened carefully to Clements's description of the symptoms before making his examination. But, apart from what he later termed "symptoms of nervous illness," Holmes could find nothing organically wrong.

"What about a brain tumor?" Clements suggested. Holmes shrugged and stuck by his original diagnosis—nerves and nothing more.

Subsequent events seemed to bear Holmes out. By March 1947 Mrs. Clements was well enough to be seen out and about with her attentive husband in the restaurants and shops of Lord Street, Southport's smartest thoroughfare. Bearing this in mind, one can well imagine Dr. Holmes's consternation when word reached him that Clements was telling friends in Manchester that Vee was still desperately ill and that it was "only a matter of time."

Clements's talent as a forecaster, like before, proved suspiciously accurate. At midnight on May 26, Holmes received a call from Clements, begging him to come around at once as his wife was dying. Holmes wasted no time. Later that night Vee Clements was admitted to the Astley Bank Nursing Home in a comatose state.

Elsewhere, Clements was making his own arrangements. He approached wealthy widow and longtime confidant Amy Stevens, asking if he could lodge with her for the duration of Vee's hospital stay. Of course, cooed Mrs. Stevens, showing him in. Much later, Amy Stevens would have to engage the services of a lawyer to protect her reputation, as a wave of scandal swept Southport linking her name with the romantic Dr. Clements. But for the time being, she was only too happy to oblige.

At the nursing home, Vee was examined by the superintendent, Dr. Andrew Brown. In the company of the matron, Mrs. Baxendale, he immediately noticed something strange about the patient's eyes—her pupils had contracted to pinpoints. Also, her skin was taking on a bluish tinge and she had trouble breathing.

Mrs. Baxendale sniffed, "Looks more like morphine poisoning to me than cerebral trouble." Dr. Brown nodded grim assent. Before departing from the nursing home that night, Brown left strict instructions that, under no circumstances, was morphine to be given to the patient, not even if prescribed by Dr. Holmes.

Despite the best attentions of everyone present Vee Clements died next morning at 9:30 without regaining consciousness. On being told, Clements immediately reiterated his theory of a cerebral tumor. Dr. Holmes was unimpressed and told Clements that he wished to conduct a postmortem to establish the cause of death. Clements agreed readily.

For some reason, in a reckless display of high-handedness, Dr. Holmes obviated the coroner's office and arranged for a postmortem to be held in the very room where Vee Clements had died. It was a course of action that later brought Holmes a stinging courtroom rebuke from the coroner, who said, "If this case had been reported to me as it might have, and ought to have been, the interests of justice would have been better served." Further commenting, the coroner added that, "to say the least, it is very disturbing."

The postmortem was carried out by Dr. James Houston, a brilliant thirty-nine-year-old pathologist at Southport Infirmary. Houston, a perfectionist who drove himself to exhaustion, was fast making a name for his work in diphtheria; he also happened to be a close friend of Dr. Robert Clements.

Before the autopsy began, Clements collared the younger man and fed him his own ideas of what had caused Vee's death. Clements was at his most beguiling. He persisted with his belief that it was a brain tumor but, for the first time, mentioned the possibility of myeloid leukemia. This was a shrewd move. Houston's ears perked up. A hematologist by speciality, any talk of blood disease was sure to grab his attention. He listened closely to what Clements had to say—after all, the older man's credentials were impeccable—and, as later events showed, plainly went into the postmortem determined to find the evidence necessary to back his friend's claims.

When Houston removed the dead woman's brain, he found no indication of a cerebral tumor. He passed these finding to Dr. Brown. Now more suspicious than ever,

Brown instructed Houston to go ahead and perform a full autopsy.

For the next two hours, James Houston conducted an almost textbook postmortem. He excised all the relevant organs, took sufficient samples of blood for analysis, made copious notes. Then the young doctor did something medically unforgivable. Whether through tiredness or a misplaced belief in his own diagnostic skills, Houston ordered the lab technician to go ahead and destroy all the organs, even though they had not yet been subjected to microscopic examination. It was criminally stupid conduct.

Back in his own laboratory, Houston hurriedly tested the blood samples and, sure enough, found what he thought to be myeloid leukemia. Satisfied, he signed the death certificate to this effect and went on to the next case.

Once again, it seemed, Robert Clements had pulled it off.

But Dr. Brown was still not convinced. Sidestepping Holmes, he followed proper procedures and took his suspicions to the local coroner, Cornelius Bolton. Bolton, appalled by Holmes's arbitrary attitude, acted swiftly, contacting the chief constable, the same Lieutenant-Colonel Harold Mighall who had attempted eight years before to stop the funeral of the third Mrs. Clements. Mighall ordered an immediate investigation.

On the evening of his wife's death, Clements dined out with longtime friends Joseph and Kathleen Milward at Rowntrees, a local restaurant. Apart from the occasional muttered reference to "poor Vee" he seemed very composed and normal. After the meal, however, Clements made a radical departure from his customary behavior. He invited his dinner guests back to his flat. At the front door he halted them and said, "I'm afraid, Joe, you are going to get a very great shock. Nobody has ever been in this flat beyond the drawing room, except you and Kathleen tonight." Clements then proceeded to demonstrate why.

He unlocked the door and led them inside. The Milwards followed, puzzled and somewhat hesitant. When Clements threw open the door of the lounge his guests could only gape.

Neither had seen such squalor.

Every room was stuffed with old and putrid food. Sprouting potatoes and rotting grapefruit lay strewn across the floor. In the kitchen, wallpaper hung in damp, foot-long shreds, dangling on to dozens of boxes packed with rancid butter and margarine. Vee Clements had crammed the pantry with countless jars of marmalade—a fetish of hers—both homemade and bought. Beneath the kitchen table someone had piled coal and twigs, then trampled soot into the bedroom where the blankets and eiderdowns were "like the back of a chimney," as Joseph Milward later testified. The lumber room defied entry because of all the junk stacked high to the ceiling. Clements sadly pointed out the mounds of newspapers, some seven years old, an ancient iron bedstead, a bicycle, hat rack, all matted with cobwebs and covered in dust.

If Clements was on a mission to demonstrate his wife's eccentricity, then he certainly succeeded. The Milwards, unable to countenance a doctor and his wife living in such filth, were stunned, reeling from the stench. Clements talked with obvious embarrassment of his wife's obsessive and slovenly behavior. He had the air of someone making a clean breast of things. The Milwards offered to help him find a housekeeper. "For God's sake get one who can cook," pleaded Clements. "I have not had a cooked meal in this house since we got married."

The Milwards proved loyal friends. The next day, while Clements was out visiting his brother, they did their best to clean up the mess at his flat. On their own admission, though, they had to stop after removing eleven sackfuls of rubbish and barely making a dent in the problem.

In the meantime the police were uncovering all sorts of interesting information about the ill-used doctor and his peculiar wife. They spoke to a woman named Mary Keefe, housekeeper to another tenant in The Promenade, who had known Vee Clements for twelve years and had often met her on the porch or in the yard. She said that Mrs. Clements frequently talked about her illness and described the symptoms, bouts of unconsciousness and weakness in the legs, but that her husband always seemed to know about these episodes in advance, advising her to go to bed early on the night the attack was due."

Mary Keefe also said that Mrs. Clements's condition had generally worsened over the past two years but especially in recent weeks when her complexion had become quite yellow. Neither did Mrs. Keefe think much of Clements's protestations that he and his wife were devoted to each other; "He was a very good actor," she said, adding, "He was teaching her very nicely."

Further fanning the flames of suspicion, another of Vee's friends told the police how Clements had tried to stop her having any contact with his wife, even to the point of removing the phone so that they could not converse.

But, most sinister of all, the police learned that Clements had been prescribing large quantities of morphine sulphate tablets for patients who did not need them. When contacted, these patients were unaware of these prescriptions and had certainly not received any of the medication.

It was this revelation that prompted Chief Constable Mighall to act. With what must have been a strange feeling of déjà vu, he gave orders for the funeral of the fourth Mrs. Clements to be stopped and a fresh autopsy conducted.

When news of this development reached Dr. James Houston, the young doctor was devastated. Certain his career was finished, he sat slumped, head in his hands, mumbling over and over again, "My God, I wish I had known this before."

That same night, Robert Clements dined out at a hotel on The Promenade, only a few yards from his flat. With him were his son, George, recently demobilized from the Navy, and his seventy-eight-year-old brother, Ernest, also a doctor. Also present was an unidentified woman acquaintance. By this time Clements knew of the impending postmortem but, if he had any inkling of the dire suspicion he was under, it did not show. According to the hotel proprietor, he seemed his usual convivial self. At the evening's conclusion, Clements walked back alone to number 20. Slowly, he climbed the stairs and entered his flat.

The next day, mourners at Christ Church were met by the vicar and told that Vee Clements's funeral service had been canceled to allow for a second postmortem. The congregation dispersed, muttering excitedly to one another. One of those most puzzled was the undertaker, a Mr. Dennison. He didn't have a clue what to do next. In order to clear up the misunderstanding, he called at Clements's flat later that morning. A wreath lay unattended on the doorstep when Dennison arrived. Not receiving an answer to his knock, Dennison let himself into the apartment. He was no stranger to the flat, having been there a few days before to remove some furniture, so was unsurprised by the appalling mess. Calling out the doctor's name, he moved from room to room, eventually entering the bedroom.

It was like no bedroom he had ever seen before. Soiled

underwear and shoes were thrown willy-nilly across two of the filthiest mattresses imaginable. A thin film of soot covered everything. As Dennison picked his way through the discarded clothing, he glanced up at the mantelpiece. A shiver iced his spine. False teeth grinned down at him. They belonged to Robert Clements. Their owner lay, fat, pale and gray-haired, on one of the beds. At first Dennison thought the doctor was asleep, then he realized that Clements was unconscious. Beside him was a note. It read:

> My dear Ernie and George—I cannot stand this diabolical insult to me. Thanks to Mr. and Mrs. Pickering for many kindnesses. Please, Ernie and George, carry on. God bless you. Always, Bertie.

He was alive but barely. Dennison ran downstairs and summoned help. An ambulance rushed Clements to the infirmary but it was too late. Robert George Clements was pronounced dead on arrival from a massive overdose of morphine. He was sixty-seven years old.

For the second postmortem on Vee Clements, the authorities took no chances. They called in Dr. W. H. Grace, a senior Home Office pathologist. With most of the vital organs missing, he faced an uphill task. Even so, he was able to satisfy himself that death was definitely not due to myeloid leukemia. Beyond that he wasn't prepared to say until he'd consulted with his colleague, Dr. J. B. Firth, director of the Home Office Forensic Laboratory at Preston. Together the two men performed forensic miracles. Working on just a short section of spine weighing less than an ounce, Firth discovered a small puncture wound, the kind made by a hypodermic syringe. Tests lasted a fortnight, but he was finally able to locate a positive reaction to the presence of morphine, 1.34 mg in the kidney and 0.8 mg in the spine. He estimated that this was but a tiny fraction of the original dose and almost certainly the cause of death.

The police, too, had been busy. They gutted the flat where Clements had lived. Among the filth they found dozens of bottles of tablets in every room. The label on one read "Phenobarbitone, one to be taken night and morning." When analyzed, the supposed sleeping tablets were found to contain three quarters of a grain of morphine sulphate. The inference was inescapable—Dr. Robert Clements had been slowly poisoning his wife over several months.

Denied the excitement of a full-scale trial, the inhabitants of Southport looked forward instead to the forthcoming inquest. It promised to be a spellbinder. But absolutely no one was expecting what happened next.

On June 2, l947, Dr. James Houston was found dead in his laboratory at Southport Infirmary. He had committed suicide by taking over three hundred times the lethal dose of sodium cyanide. He, too, left a note:

> I have for some time been aware that I have been making mistakes. I have not profited by my experience. I was convinced that Mrs. Clements died of leukemia, and accordingly destroyed the vital organs after completing my autopsy.

So now the eager public had a triple inquest to look forward to. They weren't disappointed.

The sensational story of Dr. Robert Clements drew reporters from all over England. They packed the coroner's courtroom. At times journalistic fervor threatened to get in the way of truth as wads of press money were waved at anyone connected with the case in order to get exclusive interviews. The coroner warned members of the jury to set aside any preconceived notions that they might have and listen instead to the evidence presented and make their decision on that and that alone.

The most intriguing element of that evidence was Clements's own diary. It was an odd compendium of fact and outright falsehood, and reads as though it was written for an outsider's benefit. His account of his wife's last few months are in direct contrast to those of friends. Clements's continual claims that his wife was disorientated and vague did not square with witnessed accounts of visits she and Clements made to restaurants in Southport, outings in which Vee seemed very cheerful indeed. But it was the entry for May 26, the day before her death, that revealed the biggest discrepancies. Clements's diary reads:

> Set out for a walk in the afternoon. Tea at home. After tea went for a walk to the Post Office. Vee commenced to lose voice. Losing power in her limbs. Got her home with difficulty and with fearful headache. Got her to bed, prepared tea, and Vee felt better after it. After washing up found her unconscious. Sent for Dr. Holmes.

Compare this with the sworn statement of an upstairs neighbor who saw the couple return home arm in arm, at 10:15 PM, and described Mrs. Clements as "very bright and cheerful," and in no need of assistance whatsoever. As the coroner so adroitly pointed out, less than an hour later this same woman lay unconscious and dying.

The next entry in Clements's diary was even more sinister. Referring to Vee as "an adorable wife . . . good and devoted. Never fair to herself," Clements went on to give the time of her death as 9:15 AM. In fact the records at Astley Bank Nursing Home showed that Mrs. Clements

did not die until 9:30 AM. On the surface this was an understandable slip in highly charged circumstances, until one
considers the testimony of Joseph Milward. He was most
emphatic in his assertion that Clements had called him
with the news of Mrs. Clements's death a full half hour
earlier, at 8:57 AM. And neither had the doctor seemed
greatly upset. These points told heavily with the jury. Here
they had Clements clearly expecting his wife to die and anticipating the event in the most callous fashion.

The coroner concluded three days of testimony by in-
structing the jury that, under British law, the apparent lack
of motive should play no part in their deliberations. It was
their duty to decide whether or not the death of Amy
Victoria Clements was a willful act of murder and return
their verdict accordingly.

He also clarified the situation concerning Clements. In
this case one of two verdicts was possible: either suicide
while of unsound mind, or the much rarer *felo de se* (literally self-murder, undertaken to avoid the inevitable consequences of his actions). It was a fine distinction. Suicide
implied a degree of mental imbalance; self-murder carried
no such qualification.

Coroner Bolton dealt at length with the death of Dr.
Houston. He emphasized the tragic nature of Houston's involvement in the affair. Medical records showed a long history of depression. Long before the term had ever been
invented, the young pathologist was a true workaholic.
Here, Bolton suggested, the jury might consider that the
evidence spoke for itself.

The jury took only forty-five minutes to return verdicts
as follows:

1. Amy Victoria Clements was murdered by Dr. Robert
Clements.

2. Dr. Clements committed *felo de se*.

3. Dr. Houston took his own life while the balance of his mind was disturbed.

Convicted posthumously, Robert George Clements achieved a lasting notoriety. Today such interest would be merely academic. In 1975 a bill, inspired by the Lord Lucan case, passed Parliament, restricting the power of a coroner's court to name a person as guilty of murder. Henceforth, in the eyes of the law, if you had not been tried and convicted, no one could say you were guilty.

The police decided against resurrecting the cases of Clements's three previous wives. They had nothing to gain and only the taxpayer would lose. But there were many who puzzled over why Clements decided to kill his last wife. They pointed to the fact that each of his previous victims was only eliminated when her money ran out. At her death, Vee Clements was still very well off. Her estate totalled £51,000, surely enough to keep even a satyr like Clements in relative comfort for the rest of his days.

So why do it? Most often suggested is the likelihood that Clements wanted to clear the way for further sexual conquests. But this ignores the fact that his was a lifetime devoted to adultery. Marriage to Vee had been conducted against an endless backdrop of not-so-illicit liaisons. Clements openly flaunted his latest paramour even while Vee lay sick in her bed. It is hard to imagine him wanting to disturb such a convenient status quo. There had to be another reason.

A far more compelling motive is suggested by the atrocious condition of the flat at 20 The Promenade. Vee Clements was clearly a very odd woman. Her obsessional food hoarding might be explained away by the privations of wartime, but the utter squalor and filth that investigators found can only be attributed to the crankiest of minds. For a doctor, even one as warped and sociopathic as Robert Clements, it must have been intolerable.

And there was, of course, the little matter of £51,000 to be considered.

In the end it was probably the money that swayed him. On three occasions Clements had killed and got away with it. Now in his sixties, with time running out and trapped in a sluttish marriage, he saw the chance to be rid of his obnoxious wife. For someone as ruthless as Robert George Clements, the temptation would have been too great. Living high on the hog had become a habit to him. So had murder.

4. MUSIC HATH CHARMS . . .

Watching Dr. John Hill at work in the operating theater was quite an experience. One well-heeled female patient commented, "Last thing I remember is being wheeled in . . . and seeing this gorgeous-looking guy smiling down at me. All around the sound of Beethoven thundered."

The affluent Houston-based plastic surgeon wouldn't have had it any other way. He loved the theater filled with classical music. To indulge his passion, he transported a portable stereo system with him from hospital to hospital. In this respect he was far from unique; many surgeons like music in the background while they are operating. But where Hill differed was in priorities. Given a choice between the scalpel and the gramophone, the music won hands down every time.

From his earliest days on the seventy-five-acre farm in Edcouch, South Texas, it had always been the music that came first. Piano, violin, trombone, flute, tuba, recorder— John Hill played them all with varying degrees of fluency. He and younger brother Julian practiced for hours, nonstop. It drove their mother half crazy. She didn't want any son of hers busting his ass to hold down a job in some band or orchestra, no sir; she had her sights set on better things. In one respect Myra Hill was lucky. John had a streak of greed in him wider than the Rio Grande. He wasn't stupid. Music was cool but money was better. He'd just have to find a way to subsidize his obsession. Medicine looked like the natural choice. When he reached this decision, folks around Edcouch said you could hear Myra Hill's sigh of relief clear across the border in Mexico.

In later years Hill tried to downplay his origins. He worked hard at cultivating an aura of "up from nothing' but, truthfully, family circumstances were comfortable, if strict. His parents, biblical fundamentalists, strove to instill the same beliefs in their children. John picked up the bits about guilt and Hell and eternal damnation, but the rest of it washed over him.

Friends found him difficult to understand. For such a good-looking boy—broad-shouldered, dark and tall—he had remarkably little to do with girls. They always took second place to his music and studies. Hill later claimed that he didn't lose his virginity until age twenty-six. He never quite overcame the feelings of shame that sex gave him. A knowledge of this explains much that is odd in the character of John Hill. When, years later, he finally found a woman who could fulfill him sexually, he went overboard, with tragic results.

Hill kept his nose in his books and, after graduating *summa cum laude*, attended the Baylor College of Medicine in Houston. For a wide-eyed South Texas kid in the fifties this was the big-time.

Houston was just beginning to pull itself up out of the swamp and mean something. The city had been on a building binge. Easy money from the oil boom went into skyscrapers and banks and hospitals, especially hospitals. In the Texas Medical Center, a sprawling collection of hospitals and clinics just south of downtown, Houston had a facility that was the envy of the world. Rich patients came from around the world to hand their bodies, and particularly their hearts, over to the highest-priced care available. Surgeons like Denton Cooley and Michael DeBakey were standing the medical world on its ear as they operated on a seemingly endless caseload of open-heart cases, seven or eight a day, at $1,500 an operation. Besides making themselves the wealthiest doctors alive they were also picking up the other trappings of fame: TV interviews and their faces on magazine covers. Heady stuff for any medical student, but Hill was smart enough to realize that all the best talent was going into heart surgery. He wasn't in the upper echelon, he knew that; he needed to find another field of specialization.

It didn't take him long. Houston was loaded to the gills with wealthy socialites, all hustling to outdo each other in money and status: bigger houses, bigger cars, more servants—better looks. Rich old dowagers didn't mind shelling out thousands on plastic surgery either to get rid of what nature had wrought or else add on what nature had forgotten. Most went to either New York or Los Angeles. For some reason this speciality had been overlooked by the doctors in Houston. John Hill sniffed the wind and discovered where his future lay.

But first of all he needed money, lots of it, to get himself set up. Plastic surgery, perhaps more than any other medical procedure, relies on referrals. Women gossip and women have eyes. When they see that flat-chested girl, who hardly ever got noticed before, suddenly walk in one day with a figure that Michaelangelo could not have improved on, they ask questions, fast. Pretty soon word gets around that so-and-so wields a miraculous knife. When that happens the surgeon in question is off and running. Hill knew this. He also knew that, by its very nature and cost, cosmetic plastic surgery was the reserve of the rich. He needed an introduction to the upper strata of society. Maybe a wealthy wife?

Blonde and beautiful, maybe, but Joan Robinson was light years away from being your typical social butterfly. Born the only daughter of a millionaire oil dealer, she smoked and swore like a trooper, didn't give a damn who knew it, rode horses well enough to win five world championships, and made no bones about liking men. By the time she was twenty, Joan Robinson had already been married and divorced twice. To be fair, neither marriage really stood a chance. Both husbands didn't so much acquire a wife as take on a managing partner. Ash Robinson, Joan's father, was cantankerous, interfering and very, very rich. He demanded total control of his beloved Joan and did everything in his power to ensure that he got it. But he couldn't stop Joan looking.

And look she did, that fateful night at the exclusive Cork Club in Houston's Shamrock Hotel, when first she saw Dr. John Hill, laughing and joking in the company of some socialites. According to those present, Joan's jaw almost collided with her ample bosom; she was unable to believe that anyone could be so handsome. "I want him," she told a friend. "Fix it up."

Hill proved a more than willing conquest. In no time at all, talk of marriage was in the air. When Joan presented him at the family mansion on Kirby Drive in River Oaks, old man Robinson didn't think much of his prospective third son-in-law, but gave grudging assent. Hill's parents also disapproved of the liaison. Upon learning that Joan had been twice married they shot off to Houston, Bibles in hand, ready to point out all those bits about Jezebel and Salome. Their journey was long and fruitless. The marriage of Joan Robinson to John Hill went off as planned, one of the grandest events in the crowded 1957 Houston social calendar. The bride was ecstatic. Hill was more interested in the gleaming Cadillac that Ash bought him. After their honeymoon the newlyweds moved into Ash's mansion. The old man wanted it that way. He hated Joan being out of his sight.

In short order the differences between Joan and Hill began to manifest themselves. She thrived on a diet of horse shows, gossipy cocktail parties and country clubs. Hill wanted none of that. His idea of a good time was to settle down with a rackful of classical record albums and play them one after the other late into the night.

With the arrival of their son in 1960, Joan prayed that her domestic situation would improve. It might well have done so had not the old man insisted on sticking his nose in. Ash proudly held little Robert aloft and announced that, henceforth, the baby would be known as "Boot." Old Ash doted on his grandson the same way that he had on Joan. Hill watched the spectacle from a corner, brooding and resentful. Recognizing his own impotence, he became even more isolated from his wife.

At first life on Kirby Drive was easy for the young doctor, but eventually Ash's incessant carping about having a freeloader for a son-in-law got to him. Reluctantly, in 1963, Hill joined Nathan Roth, one of Houston's top plastic surgeons, as junior partner. What should have been an auspicious occasion was marred when, a few days later, Hill's brother, Julian, also a doctor, swallowed a handful of barbiturates and killed himself. It was rumored, though never confirmed, that he was distraught over the recent breakup of a homosexual affair. Much later, Ash Robinson

would hint darkly that all was not as it seemed with the suicide of Julian Hill. The way Ash told it, John Hill had actually murdered his younger brother to keep anyone from
learning of his sexual preferences.

But all of that lay in the future. For now John Hill was
making giant strides in his practice. He hustled and he
charmed and he worked harder than anyone thought hu-
manly possible. No one could recall a more industrious
young doctor. Even so, Nathan Roth was uneasy. There
was too much conveyor belt and not enough technique.
Hill refused to heed the latest medical updates or advances,
caring only about numbers, more and more patients.
Occasionally Roth had to reprimand him for promising too
much, pointing out that they were in the business of adjust-
ment and improvements, not miracles. Hill would shrug
off these warnings and carry on churning them out. Such
high volume inevitably led to slipshod workmanship. Hot
in pursuit came the complaints. Then came the malpractice
suits. Hill couldn't have cared less about such trivia; he
had far more important fish to fry—music.

He and other similarly inclined physicians had formed
an ensemble called the Heartbeats. They played for their
own amusement and at the occasional private party. Hill
desperately wanted to play the feature instrument, piano,
but his ability never quite matched his enthusiasm and he
had to settle for the tuba. Even so, the group took over his
entire life. He organized his operating schedule so that it
didn't interfere with rehearsals. Whenever there was a conflict that he couldn't resolve, the music always won.

Despite this cavalier attitude, Hill finally began making
serious money from his practice. Not that Joan ever knew.
All he allowed her was $100 a month housekeeping. Even
though they still lived, all expenses paid, in the family
house, it wasn't anywhere near enough pocket money for a

woman of such extravagant tastes. She complained to her father. The old man's commiserations had a hollow ring to them. Having Joan on a tight financial rein ensured that his control of her would not be diminished. Joan got sympathy but not much else. In 1965, after years of pestering, Ash eventually agreed to help the couple buy a $95,000 house, just four blocks along Kirby Drive. That way Joan could maintain the pretense of independence to her friends without ever being too far from his watchful eye. To cover the down payment Ash forked over an interest-free loan of $12,000. Hill took out a mortgage for the rest.

It should have been paradise, but it didn't turn out that way. Hill's aversion to Joan festered and spread. He couldn't bear to be at home alone with her, her bad language and smoking and her lack of attendance at church. The only time friends saw them together was at social functions. In her darker moments Joan hinted to friends that, sexually, they had problems: "We don't get along too well in that department." For such a lusty woman, it must have been a demoralizing admission. John, she said sardonically, only cared for sex if it was either immoral or illegal.

In the meantime, Hill's association with Nathan Roth was also in difficulty. Their partnership limped through until 1966. By that time Roth was ready to call it a day. When the split came it degenerated into a bitterly fought battle. Roth took his case to court. Hill, never a good loser, decided to spite his ex-partner in the meanest way possible. He took a suite of offices in the same building as Roth, then did his damndest to steal away Roth's patients as well.

Hill worked like a demon. He built up his practice fast. In just his first year he grossed $168,000, a fantastic sum for those days. The cheerful office atmosphere he created for his patients spilled over to his nurses. They adored him, as well they might. Besides the obvious crushes that many had for the handsome doctor, he was also a very generous employer. Their hefty monthly checks put them among the highest paid nurses in Houston.

But back at home John Hill was still as stingy as ever. True, Joan now received $700 per month housekeeping, but she had no idea that this was a mere drop in the ocean to Hill. He told her nothing of his finances. With good reason. He had something else planned for his money.

It had always been his fantasy one day to have the perfect music room, a place where he could sit and indulge his passion in acoustical perfection, with the very best stereo equipment, even a Bösendorfer grand piano. Perhaps, one day, he might even invite the greats to come and perform for him alone. When he shared this dream with Joan, she first gave him a sidelong glance, then asked the cost. Hill shrugged his broad shoulders diffidently; $10,000 should cover it. Joan gasped. Didn't he realize they were already in hock to the bank for the $30,000 it had cost to set up his practice? Where were they going to get that kind of money from? John flashed a knowing grin and inclined his head towards the mansion just down the street.

Ash Robinson turned him down in no time flat. He'd never heard of such a dumb idea. Besides, Hill still owed him for the down payment. In a fury, Hill remortgaged his own house, paid off Ash, and used the balance to begin work on his fantasy room.

This obsession drove an even bigger wedge into the already faltering marriage. Hill's every waking thought went into the construction of his music room. Joan was relegated more and more to the background. Even worse for her was the lack of attention that Hill paid to Boot. Most days he never even saw his son except at breakfast time. Often Hill didn't come home till late at night when Boot was already asleep, and sometimes he didn't come home at all. Joan complained that Boot was growing up without a father, and it was about time that Hill did something about it. To calm Joan down Hill condescended to go with her and pick up Boot from summer camp.

It was to be the most fateful day of their lives.

Living a mile or so to the south of River Oaks, three-time divorcée Ann Kurth also decided to drive up that same day to Camp Rio Vista and collect her kids. She went alone, figuring that she would find plenty of company at the camp. Ann Kurth was not a woman who went long without company. Close to forty years old and looking like Elizabeth Taylor, she strutted her stuff that afternoon in sprayed-on jeans and T-shirt, a real head turner, even more so after taking a tumble into the lake. As she waded ashore, all of Ann's considerable charms were on full display. The guys gaped and their wives growled. Ann Kurth loved it. At some point in the afternoon she got talking to the smoothly handsome Hill. He took some photos of Ann and her three kids, promising to let her see them when they were developed.

Hill was as good as his word. A week later he showed up at Ann's place in the Memorial district. Ann, nothing if not a good hostess, invited him in. He stayed the night.

Whatever it was that Hill couldn't find with his wife he found with Ann. She coaxed him out of his sexual inertia. The resulting explosion left him besotted with her, acting like a teenager, calling at all hours of the day just to talk. Ann did nothing to dissuade him; after all, Hill, a successful surgeon, was some catch. He became a more than willing puppet on the end of her string, swept along on a tidal wave of sex, sex and more sex.

At the end of August 1968 Joan came home to find a

note. It said, "Things are not good between us, I've gone away for a few days to find myself." Miserable beyond belief, she hired an off-duty cop to track down her husband's whereabouts. It wasn't difficult. He came back with the news that Hill and Ann Kurth were definitely an item. He also gave Joan the interesting tidbit that most of Hill's possessions were in the trunk of his Cadillac; she might find something of interest there. The next day, with a friend standing guard, Joan rifled the contents of the trunk. In it she found receipts for presents, cleared checks to all kinds of women, proof that the money he had studiously avoided giving her was going to support a veritable harem. Joan rushed home in tears.

Upon learning that Hill had rented a small bachelor apartment, Joan swallowed her pride and went calling. Her reception was frosty. Hill loftily explained that Ann completely dominated his life; he couldn't come home even if he wanted to. Over the next few weeks Hill gave ample evidence of his infatuation. He hawked Ann all over Houston. So blatantly did he behave that the Heartbeats were forced to take Hill to one side and suggest that it might be best for all concerned if he didn't bother showing up any more. The amorous doctor had become an embarrassment, a liability to them. This ostracism hit Hill hard, worse than upsetting his wife, but he didn't stop his relentless pursuit of Ann Kurth. He couldn't.

Strange as it may seem, throughout this entire fiasco construction on the fabulous music room still went ahead. By November 1968 Hill had blown $75,000 on the venture, in the belief that one day the house on Kirby Drive would be his again. Ever the optimist, in mid-November he served divorce papers on Joan.

When Ash Robinson heard this development, the old man decided that enough was enough.

Hill got the telephone call at his apartment. He listened in stone-faced silence to what Ash had to say. Those who knew Ash thought it probably ran something along the lines of, "Get your ass over here this minute or I'll make damn sure that you never see your son again!"

Whatever it was that Ash used to bludgeon Hill into submission, it worked. Hill drove to Kirby Drive immediately. Once there, he signed a strange document, written out in Ash's own hand, begging a reconciliation with Joan and asking her forgiveness for his transgressions. After that came a promise to sign over his interest in the house and to increase the monthly stipend to $1,000 a month. Just to rub it in, Ash bullied Hill into settling $7,000 on Joan right away. Oh yes, and he also had to drop any notion of legal separation.

And so the prodigal husband returned. Joan threw a reconciliation party, just a small do, with a couple of friends. It generated into a near wake. Hill was morose and didn't say much to anyone. He had other things on his mind.

Later, around midnight, the phone beside Ann Kurth's bed rang. She let it ring several times before answering. It was Hill. Any chance that he could see her next day for lunch?

John Hill was trapped. On the one hand he needed the security that Joan, or more accurately Ash, could provide, but he couldn't leave Ann alone. She could twist him every which way but loose. The couple resumed their illicit liaison. Piece by piece, Ann Kurth took over his life, showing up at the office, demanding to see his accounts. Anyone who got in her way received a torrent of abuse. The upheaval reached such a pitch that Hill began missing appointments. In the end his nurses, their loyalty tested to breaking point, wouldn't even put him on the schedule.

But still John Hill couldn't or wouldn't break free.

The attempt to salvage his marriage became less and less important to him. Some indication of where his priorities laid can be gauged by the events of Christmas Day 1968. Hill passed the early part of the morning with Joan and Boot. Then he made his usual excuse—patients to see—and left. The remainder of that day he spent carousing in a southwest Houston motel with Ann Kurth.

Joan wasn't dumb. She confided to friends that Hill was still cheating on her, and he was still plowing money into that music room. So far it had cost them $100,000, more than the original cost of the house. Joan cursed. Playing second fiddle to another woman was bad enough; losing her husband to a goddamn room was unbearable.

It became all too apparent that Hill just couldn't be bothered with his family. On St. Valentine's Day 1969 he visited Ann's house, loaded down with presents for her and the kids. Back at the gloom-filled house on Kirby Drive, Joan was left to explain to Boot why Daddy wasn't there, and why he hadn't spent a dime on either of them.

Joan did a great job of papering over the cracks. Whenever friends visited, she didn't mind showing off the music room. Guests were awestruck. Even by the flashy standards of River Oaks this was opulence on a hitherto unseen scale. Hill's vision had translated itself into a vast ballroom, hung with rich satins and brocade. Joan wryly referred to it as "our own little Versailles." She had a point. Crystal chandeliers and a huge candelabra glistened in the reflected light. The walls were lined with gold panels. Behind these Hill kept his vast collection of records and instruments. A movie screen appeared at the touch of a button. And, of course, there was the Bösendorfer piano. But pride of place went to the $20,000 sound system: it contained four miles of wiring and 108 speakers and delivered the music in Wagnerian-sized chunks. Hill would sit entranced for hours.

With the completion of his music room, Hill's resentment of Joan went into overdrive. He didn't want anything to do with her. His mind began working. Springtime in Houston is a season of sudden violent storms. Secluded in the cloistered magnificence of his music room, John Hill knew this. He also knew that, out there on the horizon, his own particular storm clouds were beginning to gather.

The first signs of impending disaster came on a March night in 1969. Joan was at home, entertaining two girl-friends from Dallas and making excuses for her absent husband. As usual, Hill was at the hospital, or so he claimed. Later that evening he showed up, effusive and full of bonhomie, most unlike him. He also had some pastries which he insisted that the ladies enjoy. Hill doled the pastries out carefully. Take the chocolate one, he told Joan; it's your favorite. Eager to please, Joan did as she was told.

Two days later the strange pastry ritual was repeated. And, again, Hill was insistent that Joan have the chocolate éclair.

Another two days after that, on Thursday, Hill showed up an hour late for dinner at a small stud farm that Joan owned. Once again he came bearing gifts—more pastries. By this time Joan was ready to tell her husband what he could do with his pastries, especially when his beeper summoned him to the hospital as it did most nights at this time.

Next day she and Hill had a battle royal. It ended with Hill backing out of the driveway in his Cadillac, Joan chasing him, yelling fit to bust. Even on Kirby Drive, where the houses were about a football field apart, neighbors couldn't help but hear her frantic cry, "You've blown it,

John. You've just lost your wife, your son and that goddamn music room."

Later that night Hill, displaying the almost supernatural self-control that was his trademark, returned to the house, acting for all the world as though nothing had happened. Not only that, but he gave Joan a pill to calm her nerves. Then they went to bed.

All next day Joan felt groggy. By evening she was well enough to invite some friends over. Some of her feistiness had returned as well. A bizarre bridge game took place in the music room with Joan passing handwritten messages to her playing companions, detailing Hill's infidelities. At the other end of the room Hill was too engrossed in his music to notice, or so he tried to pretend. Just before the guests left they witnessed an extraordinary *rapprochement* between the estranged couple—John and Joan Hill were dancing romantically together! All the guests could do was shake their heads. None of this made any sense.

The next morning, Sunday, Joan felt really ill, sick to her stomach. Hill told friends that it was a virus, the flu possibly. Over the next forty-eight hours Joan Hill, normally the most robust of people, became sicker than anyone had ever seen her before. Early on Tuesday morning Hill summoned the maid, Effie Green, and ordered her to take care of Joan. While Hill went off to a tuba recital, poor Effie did her best to clean off the feces that Joan had been lying in for hours. She tried hauling Joan into the bathroom. Before they could reach it, Joan lost control of her bowels completely. "I don't want to die," she kept moaning.

"You ain't gonna die," soothed Effie. But the blue in Joan's face and her nonstop shivering must have made the elderly maid wonder.

Hill was summoned back to the house. He loaded Joan

into his car and took her to the hospital, except that he
didn't take her to the Texas Medical Center, which was fifteen minutes away and had the best doctors in America.
Instead he set out for Sharpstown Hospital, a small neighborhood hospital in which he had a financial interest. The
eleven miles' journey took him three quarters of an hour.
Joan's mother, also in the car, couldn't believe how slowly
her son-in-law was driving. Later she would come to wonder if such dilatory progress had not been intentional.

At Sharpstown, Joan Hill was placed in the care of Dr.
Walter Bertinot who had only ever seen her on a couple of
occasions; he was surprised when Hill said that his wife
had specifically requested that he attend her. Bertinot
checked Joan's blood pressure and found it dangerously
low, 60/40. If he couldn't increase the volume there was a
very real possibility that she would die of shock. His initial
diagnosis was dysentery, possibly caused by salmonella
food poisoning. Over the next ten hours he saw Joan
weaken in front of him. That night at nine o'clock a call
went out, "Get John Hill here quickly." Two hours later the
doctor finally showed up.

He wasn't able to do much except watch. When tired of
that, Hill went for a nap in a nearby room. Joan Hill's tor-
ment came to an end at 2:30 AM. One last hemorrhage
spewed blood from her mouth and then she died. She was
just thirty-eight years of age.

Aroused from his sleep, Hill became hysterical. He
turned in quite a performance, sobbing and prostrating
himself across Joan's bloated, blood-soaked body. In the
end he had to be assisted from the room.

Under such circumstances any grieving spouse might
be forgiven for actions which are later deemed to be inap-
propriate, but the fact remains that, over the next few
hours, John Hill engaged in a variety of practices which

were questionable at best and, quite possibly, much, much worse.

Under Texas law an autopsy must be performed on any patient who dies within twenty-four hours of admission to a hospital. Before the coroner can release the body he must be satisfied as to cause of death. Hill knew this but immediately called a firm of local undertakers and asked them to collect Joan's body. This they duly did at 6:00 AM, less than four hours after death. Another forty-five minutes later and they were at work.

In Texas it was by no means uncommon for autopsies to be carried out at funeral parlors, but when Sharpstown pathologist Dr. Arthur Morse showed up at 10:00 AM he was shocked to learn that the body had been drained of its fluids. Embalming fluid had pushed out the blood before it, along with the best opportunity of finding out what had killed Joan Hill. Morse did the best he could. The autopsy concluded at 11:30 AM. Morse could not find any obvious cause of death but, from the almost maroon color of the pancreas, hazarded that the most likely possibility was pancreatitis. Thus was born the first opinion as to what had killed Joan Hill. In the fullness of time there would be several others.

When the undertakers contacted Hill for any last-minute instructions, he seemed indifferent except on one point. He didn't want Joan taking any jewelry to the grave with her. The dress was decoration enough. The undertakers assured him that this would be done.

Despite John Hill's best efforts to keep Joan's death low-key, the Houston grapevine was already humming.

How could Joan Hill who, only days before had been looking marvelous and full of vitality, die so suddenly? It just didn't add up.

Someone thinking along these very same lines was Ash

Robinson. The old man took it hard. Joan had meant the world to him. And now she was gone. There had to be a reason . . .

Giving his suspicions a shove in the right direction was a friend of Joan's who had visited Hill, offering condolences. Expecting a bereaved husband the woman was appalled to find Hill and some cronies curled up in front of the movie screen, shrieking with laughter at a Laurel and Hardy film. In disgust she stormed down the road to Ash's house and relayed her findings. Their conversation lasted well into the night. By its conclusion Ash Robinson knew what had to be done.

Next morning, the day of the funeral, he showed up at the district attorney's office and said, "I have reason to believe that my son-in-law murdered my only child." He ran off his list of reasons and Assistant DA McMaster had to admit that they did sound fishy. He called Houston county coroner, Dr. Joseph Jachimczyk, with a request for him to attend the funeral and see what he thought.

Jachimczyk's first course of action was to call Sharpstown Hospital and bawl them out for the improper way they had conducted themselves. Then he gave Morse a royal dressing-down. Microscopic examination of sections taken from the pancreas of Joan Hill disclosed that the reddening of the pancreas had actually occurred postmortem, by the pancreas feeding on itself. Morse, acutely embarrassed by this finding, now had to admit that he didn't have a clue as to the cause of death. Jachimczyk went on to ask what specimens remained. Morse mumbled something about sections of liver, pancreas, kidney and a small amount of stomach contents. Jachimczyk ordered them to be sent to his office right away.

Afterward Jachimczyk went to the chapel where the body of Joan Hill lay. Any hopes that he could carry out this visit surreptitiously went unfulfilled. The River Oaks bush telegraph began beating like a drum. Soon everyone knew that something was up.

Joan Hill was laid to rest at a cemetery near her beloved stud farm. The funeral was a lavish, glitzy affair. Not only do wealthy Texans like to live in style but they die that way, too. Ash Robinson was making one of his rare visits to church. He varied his stony gaze between the casket holding his daughter's body and his son-in-law. Driving away from the cemetery, Hill insisted on being in the same car as Ash. The two men didn't speak. Ash Robinson had already made up his mind. He told his wife, "If the law doesn't get that sonofabitch, I will."

True to his word, Ash pestered the daylights out of the DA's office until he got action. He wanted to know what Jachimczyk really thought. Having examined the same specimens as Morse, Jachimczyk concluded that death was the result of acute hepatitis, probably viral in origin. Robinson took this diagnosis to a doctor friend of his. He stated that viral hepatitis was rarely fatal within two to three days; it was a much longer degenerative kind of disease. Considering how well Joan had been just days before her death, the doctor considered it most unlikely that she could have succumbed to this illness.

All fired up with this knowledge, Ash commissioned ex-DA Frank Briscoe, now in private practice, to uncover evidence of foul play. Briscoe approached Jachimczyk, asking if hepatitis could be caused by injection. Jachimczyk conceded the possibility but argued that there was nothing to suggest that this had happened. Briscoe reported this information to Ash Robinson and was told to keep looking.

The unflinching drive and supercilious vanity that had propelled John Hill to the top of his profession concealed

the fact that, at times, he could be extraordinarily stupid.
Never was this lack of common sense more amply demonstrated than when, just three months after the death of
Joan, he married Ann Kurth. Ash Robinson heard the news
and cackled with glee. He called Briscoe. This was it. Now
they had a motive. Ash kept up his badgering and finally
the DA's office gave him the grand jury investigation he
was after.

In the meantime, Ash did everything in his power to
wreck Hill's practice. He criticized his son-in-law from
one end of Houston to the other and called him a murdering sonofabitch who, by rights, should be sitting in the
electric chair at Huntsville State Prison. It worked. The
flow of patients to Hill's surgery slowed to a trickle. Worse
still, he was subpoenaed by the grand jury. They wanted
him to submit to a lie detector. Hill, who had not bothered
to hire a lawyer lest it be misinterpreted as an admission of
guilt, declined. But he would take a sodium pentothal test,
the so-called truth serum. Reluctantly the grand jury
agreed. Hill came through the exam with flying colors. So
well, in fact, that the grand jury decided that there was no
case to answer and threw it out.

Mightily disgruntled by this turn of events, Ash demanded another autopsy, this time using the best pathologist in America. He made inquiries and learned that the
current bearer of this title was the illustrious chief medical
examiner of New York, Dr. Milton Helpern. Really piquing
Ash's curiosity was the major role that Helpern had played
in getting another doctor, Carl Coppolino, convicted of
wife murder. Ash saw a lot of parallels in the two cases and
convinced himself that this time he had the right man.
Rumor had it that he paid Helpern close to $12,000 to
make the trip down to Texas. Whatever the cost, Ash reck-

oned he was getting his money's worth and that was all that mattered.

When Hill heard of this latest development he did the only sensible thing: he hired a lawyer. Not just any lawyer but Richard Haynes, known to his friends and his enemies (and he had plenty of both) as "Racehorse." It was an inspired move. Short and stocky, "Racehorse" Haynes liked to come off as just another good ole boy, but beneath the homespun exterior sizzled one of the best legal minds in not just Texas, but anywhere. First off, Haynes told Hill: Assemble your own battery of doctors. Have them on hand when Helpern performs the autopsy, just to protect your own interests.

With much media pomp and a considerable amount of fanfare, Helpern swept into Ben Taub Hospital. If anyone could find anything untoward it would be Milton Helpern. As soon as the coffin lid was pried off, Helpern bent over. Immediately his trained eye lighted on an obvious irregularity. Chunks of dried mud lay in the casket beside the body. Helpern frowned. The conclusion was inescapable—the casket of Joan Robinson Hill had already been opened.

Dr. Jachimczyk, who was present, spoke with the undertakers and learned that, three days after the funeral, John Hill had obtained a certificate allowing disinterment of the body. His reason was that he wanted to reclaim an item of jewelry which had been inadvertently buried with the body. Clearly this didn't square with Hill's insistence that Joan be buried *sans* adornment. Before speculation in the mortuary got entirely out of hand, Helpern quickly noted the total absence of anything to suggest that the body had been tampered with in any way.

Helpern conducted his autopsy with the meticulousness born of countless repetition, unlike the previous autopsy which had been perfunctory at best. The stomach was still intact, unexamined; this was remarkable, considering the likelihood that Joan Hill had died from something she ingested. Helpern tutted his disapproval. Later that disapproval turned to outright disbelief—the heart was missing! And so was the brain!

Dr. Morse, by now cringing from embarrassment, admitted that he had removed the heart for closer examination and neglected to return it for burial with the remains. He also owned up to the whereabouts of the brain. It was in the trunk of his car, parked outside! Shamefacedly, Morse brought in the jar containing Joan Hill's brain for inspection. Helpern, who by this time must have felt grave misgivings about the much-vaunted Texas medical system, examined the brain and thought he detected traces of meningitis, but declined to list that as the direct cause of death. Seven and a half hours after he began, Helpern concluded the autopsy, took his sections and his slides, and flew back to New York, promising his report would be forthcoming.

While Ash fumed and fulminated over Helpern's perceived procrastination, he was doubtless overjoyed to learn that things between Hill and his new wife were sliding downhill fast. They were fighting constantly. When it came to marital disputes, Ann was more than capable of holding her own. She ably demonstrated this during one violent quarrel by delivering a perfect right cross that broke Hill's nose. The doctor drove to a nearby hospital and amazed a group of awestruck medical students by standing in front of a mirror and setting the break himself.

Hill's domestic upheaval deteriorated to the point that he showed up at his lawyer's office, insisting on a divorce from Ann. Haynes gulped and swallowed a few times, then cleared his throat to speak. Was Hill stark raving mad? No sooner had he lost one wife, than he had acquired another, and now he wanted to get shut of her as well! Did he have some kind of death wish? Hill was adamant. Go ahead and serve the papers. Haynes explained that, under Texas law, a wife cannot testify against her husband. Given Ann's recent behavior, if Hill went ahead and filed for divorce, she could end up being a star witness for the prosecution. None of this made the slightest difference to Hill. He arrogantly dismissed Haynes's advice, emphatic that nothing would come of the judicial probings.

Around this time a further complication was introduced into the already tangled web of circumstances surrounding the death of Joan Hill. Another doctor declared that he was unable to find any traces of meningitis in the spinal cord and raised the intriguing question—had the brain been switched? This latest bombshell was gobbled up by the eager Houston public who followed the John Hill soap opera avidly in their newspapers. This was better than television any day.

At long last Helpern came back to Texas to deliver his conclusion. First, he dismissed any suggestion that the brain had been switched. He still could not determine the exact cause of death but offered "an acute inflammation of some sort," adding, "most likely by way of the alimentary tract." Helpern was implying, without being specific, that Joan Hill had been poisoned. He concluded his testimony with a scathing condemnation of the medical treatment that Joan had received, both from her husband and from the staff at Sharpstown Hospital. In his view their neglect had "aggravated a situation which proved fatal."

While none of this was the outright proof of wrongdoing that Ash Robinson wanted, it did give the DA's office something to work on. They scoured their law books for precedent and found exactly what they were looking for— an obscure charge termed "murder by omission," in effect, causing death by deliberate neglect. If they couldn't nail John Hill for what he had done, then maybe they could bag him for what he hadn't?

Less than twelve months after the death of his first wife, Hill received the divorce from Ann that he so earnestly wanted. Sure enough, within twenty-four hours Ann Kurth was in front of the grand jury, spilling the beans. She testified under oath that Hill had admitted killing Joan. Furthermore, Ann claimed that he had tried to kill her as well.

It took the best part of a year to bring Hill to trial. The prosecution, aware that their case rested almost solely on the testimony of Ann Kurth, petitioned that she be allowed to give evidence. Judge Hooey was hesitant and agreed only on the proviso that he might stop her proof at any time. Over defense objections Ann told of finding three petri dishes—the kind used in laboratories—in Hill's apartment just one week before Joan Hill died. She said, "They had something red in them." When Hill suddenly came in he became angry and shooed her from the room. He explained that it was "just an experiment." The next day Ann spotted some pastries in the refrigerator. Hill told her not to eat them.

Ann went on to describe an incident in which she claimed Hill tried to kill her, first in a car crash and then immediately afterward with a syringe. When asked by the defense how she knew that the syringe was harmful—after all, might it not have been a sedative following the traumatic incident?—Ann replied triumphantly, "Because he told me how he had killed Joan with a needle."

Haynes came off his seat, hollering "Mistrial!" at the top of his lungs. He got his wish. After due consideration Judge Hooey threw the case out on the grounds that the defense had not had an opportunity to prepare themselves against this direct accusation of murder.

In trying to condemn Hill, Ann Kurth seriously overplayed her hand. If, as she alleged, the murder attempt took place just four weeks into a nine-month marriage, why had she stayed with a man who had tried to kill her? Ann claimed to have been frightened into immobility, but everyone who knew the lady found this hard to swallow. The whole scenario had an air of unreality. The prosecutors certainly thought so. They just shook their heads and went back to the drawing board.

Any mistrial always favors the defendant; it sours the prosecution and quite often leads to a dismissal of all charges. Hill thought he was home free and decided to celebrate. He did it in just about the worst possible way—he got married again.

A mere four months after the mistrial, Connie Loesby became the third Mrs. Hill. She had been a good friend to Hill during the pretrial hoopla, helping his case along by providing legwork and enthusiasm. Hill must have wondered where Connie had been all his life. Quiet, the stay-at-home type, and, yes, a passion for music every bit as fervent as his own. The two lived a low-profile life in the big house on Kirby Drive, seemingly happy with each other, both intent on rebuilding Hill's shattered career.

He read more, went to conventions, learned the latest innovations in plastic surgery. In fact, he did all the things that his first partner, Nathan Roth, had accused him of shirking. Ironically, he and Connie were on their way back from just such a convention in Las Vegas on Sunday, September 24, 1972, when the final chapter in the extraordinary life of John Hill reached its conclusion.

They had arrived at Houston Airport and taken a cab into River Oaks. While Hill paid off the cabdriver in the driveway, Connie ran to the front door, eager to see her twelve-year-old stepson. She rang the doorbell. No one came. A minute later, through a glass panel, Connie could make out the shape of a hooded figure. She laughed. This was probably one of Boot's practical jokes. Prepared to play along, Connie smiled as the door opened. In a flash the hooded stranger reached out and yanked her inside, growling, "This is a robbery."

Hill was only a pace behind. He rushed in, threw Connie out of harm's way and went for her attacker. Connie ran, screaming, toward a neighbor's house. As she did, three shots in quick succession rang out behind her. When the police and neighbors reached the house, John Hill was lying dead on the floor. In another room they found Hill's mother, Myra, and son, Boot, both bound and gagged.

It was obvious that the killer had been waiting for Hill. His mumbled comment to Connie about this being a "robbery" was borne out by the theft of Hill's briefcase and wallet, but everything else smacked of a thoroughly professional and well-planned assassination. After shooting Hill, the killer had taped up his eyes, nose and mouth. This way, if the bullets failed to do their job, then it was a certainty that John Hill would drown in his own blood. Afterward the intruder had tossed his hood, a green pillowcase with eyeholes cut out, onto the ground beside the body.

The police had precious little to go on but underlying all that they did was a deep suspicion that Ash Robinson had paid for the death of his son-in-law. It was a charge they dared not make. The old man was too powerful and too rich. Instead the police pursued other, more orthodox inquiries, and wondered if they might not lead back to the other house on Kirby Drive.

A week after the murder they got their first break. Behind some nearby bushes an officer discovered what looked to be the murder weapon, a .38-caliber revolver. Ballistics experts checked it with a bullet found next to Hill's body. It matched. A serial number check produced a bizarre coincidence—the gun used to kill John Hill had been registered to another doctor.

The doctor in question lived in the small East Texas town of Longview, and was far from pleased by the arrival of two Houston police officers at his house. Some careful questioning revealed that the doctor maintained an unusually flamboyant lifestyle, with a particular fondness for prostitutes. It turned out that one, a girl he knew as "Dusty," had stolen his gun while he was in the bath recovering from a particularly rigorous bout between the sheets.

The police had no problems learning that "Dusty" was actually Marcia McKittrick, a Dallas prostitute. Where the difficulty lay was in locating her. Finally, more than six months after the murder, they picked up her "minder," a long-time pimp named Bobby Vandiver. Under a high-pressure grilling and the promise of just a twelve-year sentence Vandiver admitted getting the gun from Marcia McKittrick and killing Hill with it. But, he claimed, it had all been set up. He'd been hired by a middle-aged Houston housewife, Lilla Paulus; she was the one who had arranged the killing. Vandiver said he'd been paid $3,500 for the contract. He also said that Hill often carried anywhere up to $30,000 when he traveled; this explained why he stole the briefcase and wallet. In fact, Hill only had $700 on him at the time of his death, much to the hired killer's chagrin.

On Vandiver's say-so, Lilla Paulus was taken into custody and slapped with a conspiracy-to-murder charge. At about the same time, police picked up Marcia McKittrick. She corroborated Vandiver's story and also claimed to have met Ash Robinson. She, too, was charged with the murder of John Hill.

Just when the prosecution thought everything was all sewn up, fate played a wicked hand. Days before Bobby Vandiver was due to stand trial, he was involved in an altercation at a Longview bar and shot to death by a police officer. There seemed to be no connection whatsoever between this incident and the Hill case.

With their star witness dead, the prosecution turned their attention to Marcia McKittrick. She made a deal and settled for ten years on the proviso that she testify against Lilla Paulus.

To see fifty-four-year-old Lilla Paulus in court was a wondrous sight. Homely and smiling, she did her best to come off like Grandma Moses. But the police knew better. Lilla had a record going back to the forties, mostly convictions for prostitution when she'd run a whorehouse in Galveston. For the last twenty years she'd been married to a big-time Houston bookie with some very shady connections. Lilla was a woman who moved easily on the fringes and, occasionally, deep within the Houston underworld.

Most of this information had to be kept from the jury but what they heard from Lilla's own daughter, Mary Jo, was more than enough for them to make up their minds about Lilla Paulus. Mary Jo told of hearing her mother mention Ash Robinson's willingness to pay for a hit on John Hill; she had also seen Ash talking to Lilla on several occasions, once giving her a diagram of the house on Kirby Drive. According to Mary Jo, Lilla was paid $25,000 to arrange the contract killing. But the clincher came when, in a hesitant voice, Mary Jo revealed how her mother had coerced her into prostitution at the age of four. In a few simple sentences Mary Jo stripped all the contrived homeliness from Lilla Paulus and revealed her as the callous and calculating woman that she really was. Largely on the strength of her own daughter's testimony, Lilla Paulus was found guilty and sentenced to thirty-five years in prison.

For some reason the authorities never proceeded against Ash Robinson. Only a civil action brought him into court. It was filed in 1977 by the Hill family, including Connie and Boot, and alleged wrongful death. Ash hobbled to the stand on his walking cane and swore impassionedly to his grandson that he had nothing to do with the death of his father. Every answer was punctuated by staccato raps of the cane against the floor.

This time Mary Jo Paulus refused to repeat her testimony. Lilla, not unnaturally, took the Fifth Amendment and said nothing.

Which left Marcia McKittrick.

A polygraph test decided that she was being truthful when she said Ash Robinson had caused the death of John Hill. A similar test showed that Ash was being truthful when he said he hadn't; this outcome probably reveals more about the inaccuracy of polygraphs than it does about either person. Whatever the machine said, Ash Robinson was vindicated of complicity in the death of his son-in-law and allowed to go free.

So far as the courts were concerned, the extraordinary events surrounding the life and times of Dr. John Hill were over. Now it was time for the main participants to get on with the rest of their lives.

Connie Hill did just that. She remarried and took her chances in Houston, bringing up stepson Boot as best she could.

Ann Kurth set up a dress shop in central Texas.

In February 1985, at the age of eighty-seven, Ash Robinson died.

A bizarre footnote to this saga was provided by Ann Kurth. She emerged from seclusion with the startling claim that John Hill wasn't dead at all; it had all been an elaborate hoax. The cunning doctor had arranged his own demise using an impostor, changed his appearance through plastic surgery, then escaped to Guadalajara, Mexico where he was carrying on much as before. How can she be so sure that Hill is still alive?

Simple.

Every now and then the music-mad medico calls her up on the telephone. He doesn't say anything but he does play Rachmaninoff down the line . . . just for her.

5. A TASTE FOR MURDER

When it comes to motivation, most doctors who willfully destroy human life are no different from other murderers. Richard Kuklinski, the mafia hitman who boasted of a rubout list that ran into three figures, might well have derided Marcel Petiot's* methods as needless extravagance, but he would have empathized with the little Frenchman's grasping attention to the bottom line. For these two entrepreneurs, murder was a profitable business, nothing more. Similarly, the New Hampshire schoolteacher Pamela Smart could well have been joined at the hip, figuratively speaking, to Charles Friedgood. Both were highly sexed, both felt themselves to be trapped in inconvenient marriages, and both took drastic steps to remedy their situations. At the risk of sounding crass, all the above are what we might term "normal" murderers; the motive is clear and discernible, and some benefit accrues to the perpetrator.

*See chapter 9.

But what on earth are we to make of the doctor who goes bad for no apparent reason?

In recent years, there has been an epidemic of health care professionals prepared to dispatch patients just for the hell of it. This is the most dangerous medical murderer of all, because it means that every one of us is at risk. For some reason, this phenomenon seems to disproportionately afflict nurses—Donald Harvey in Ohio and New Jersey's Charles Cullen are just two candidates for the role of America's most prolific "angel of death," while Britain's deadliest nurse is a woman, Beverly Allitt—but, when it comes to relieving patients of their earthly concerns, none of these killers, as evil as they were, can approach the truly appalling Dr. Harold Shipman.

Between 1974 and 1998 this meek-mannered, almost nondescript, middle-aged Englishman killed an estimated 254 patients—and possibly more; the exact number will never be known—by injecting them with diamorphine. Most of his victims were plucked from the battalions of adoring elderly women who flocked to his surgery. At Shipman's trial in 1999, where he was imprisoned for life, the prosecutor said that "he [the defendant] must have found the drama of taking life to his taste," and it's hard to dispute that statement. Toward the end of his murderous career, it's true that Shipman did line his pockets by forging the odd will or two—ironically, it was this greed that led to his downfall—but overwhelmingly he was a thrill killer, someone who enjoyed the power of life and death over his victims. And like other slipshod or dubious medical practitioners covered in this book, he had not acted in a vacuum; in fact, his career was littered with muttered accusations and knowing winks. Many of his peers sensed something was wrong—that suspiciously high ratio of self-certified cremation authorizations was always a cause for concern—but once again the medical profession demonstrated its oxymoronic attitude to self-regulation. In Shipman's case, as the ranks closed and lips remained sealed, he continued killing at a phenomenal rate that peaked at almost forty victims per year.*

In a grotesque fluke of timing, just a few years after Shipman switched on his murderous conveyor belt in England, across the Atlantic an unwitting disciple set out on a broadly similar path. He, too, disposed of patients with malevolent and gleeful efficiency, and like Shipman, this young doctor had been branded a rogue practitioner from early on. Still that didn't prevent him from finding employment in hospitals and training schools. There is an old medical maxim that doctors get to bury their mistakes. Often they don't even need to bother. For as the following makes clear, there are plenty of others willing to wield the shovels for them.

The technicians on the Adams County paramedics team based in Quincy, Illinois had harbored doubts about the new guy right from day one. Sure, they were used to sick or gallows humor—in a job as mentally tough as theirs it came with the territory—but there were times when Michael Swango's idea of a joke really churned the stomach. The really serious alarm bells started clanging on July 14,1984, one month after he joined the team. That was the day when Swango and his fellow paramedics crowded around the TV in their quarters as graphic coverage of what became known as the San Ysidro Massacre flashed across the screen. When James Huberty, a recently dismissed security guard, stormed a local McDonald's and blasted twenty people into eternity before shooting himself, it made for some harrowing footage. Yet Swango was

*On January 13, 2004, Shipman hanged himself in his cell at Wakefield Prison.

chortling away like he was watching *Happy Days*. At one point, unable to contain his excitement, he leapt from his seat to crank the volume, hollering at the top of his lungs for others to come and share his enjoyment. Later that day, quieter and more reflective, the young newcomer was overheard to rue the fact that "every time I think of a good idea, somebody beats me to it."

He had other weird traits, too, like his fondness for eating dinner in the middle of the night, and the way he would often go twenty-four hours without hitting the sack, not because of some emergency, just because he didn't need to sleep the way normal people did. All these quirks and more, the other crew members became used to, but the one characteristic they couldn't stomach was Swango's fascination with violence. He seemed consumed by it. During quiet periods on the shift, he would entertain his reluctant colleagues by fabricating grisly 911 scenarios. His "ultimate call" for the team was one where the paramedics would rush to a scene just in time to see a gasoline trailer truck plow into a crippled school bus, blowing scores of children to kingdom come. On another occasion, when the topic of conversation shifted to serial killers, he became almost evangelical, blurting out to a coworker: "I really admire those guys, going round the country killing people." Then he grinned. It was that smile, open and broad with the twinkly blue eyes, that made Swango so difficult to assess. It underscored every outlandish utterance. Charismatic joker or just plain spooky? Most settled for the latter and gave the handsome oddball a wide berth.

On one point the technicians were united: Michael Swango was damn good at his job. When it came to medical knowledge and emergency expertise, he could run rings round all of them. Only to be expected, really, since the thirty-year-old ex-marine had already qualified as a doctor in Ohio and had taken this paramedic job purely as a stopgap while his Illinois license was being processed.

He didn't try to lord it over his teammates; he always came across as one of the guys. When they brought in cakes, cookies and candy for everyone to share, a few days later he would reciprocate. The first indications that something might be amiss with Swango's culinary contributions came at 7:30 on the morning of September 14, 1984, when he showed up with an assortment of freshly baked doughnuts for breakfast. The other four duty paramedics fell on them hungrily. Over the next hour, they fell ill one by one. Their symptoms were identical: stomach cramps and nausea, followed by dizziness, then uncontrollable retching. Each vomited so hard they had to go home. Except Swango. He seemed blissfully immune to the mystery ailment.

As painful and uncomfortable as the sudden illness undoubtedly was, it did no lasting harm to any of the paramedics, and the next evening, one of those affected, Brent Unmisig, had recovered sufficiently to accompany Swango on routine duty at a local high school football game. As halftime approached, Swango announced that he was thirsty and disappeared to buy a cola. When he returned he tossed Unmisig a Coke. He gratefully chugged it down. Before long he was suffering a bilious rerun of the day before. Swango, solicitous as always, drove his partner home, where he remained bed-bound for three days.

Two such occurrences in twenty-four hours were decidedly odd; especially as Swango had been present at both and affected by neither. Unmisig, mindful of his rookie status—he'd only joined the team on the day of the doughnut incident—was hesitant at first about sharing his suspicions about Swango, but gradually he won over his colleagues. A tacit agreement was reached that Michael Swango should come with a government health warning. In the future, whenever he offered to buy a drink for his colleagues or proffered any kind of food, it was firmly declined. Swango's pariah status kept everyone on their toes. But it failed to stem the flow of suspicious incidents.

One paramedic, believing he was on safe ground when Swango offered to fetch a couple cans of soda from a vending machine, would learn that Swango's brand of waitering came at a high price. As the can was handed to him, he noticed that the ring-pull had been yanked back. When he confronted Swango about this, that million-watt smile beamed right back at him, accompanied by an innocent shrug of the shoulders. Despite all the rumors, and against his gut instinct, the paramedic took a sip. It tasted okay. Thirty minutes later he was doubled over in agony and being rushed home. The Quincy bug had struck again.

For the paramedics, this was an incident too far. Action was called for. Biding their time until Swango was out on an emergency call, they opened up his locker. Nestling inside the bag that accompanied Swango almost everywhere was a bottle of Terro Ant Killer. When the paramedics read the label, they got a chill—the active ingredient was arsenic. A reference book told them all they needed to know.

Virtually tasteless when mixed with food or drink, arsenic was for centuries the toxin of choice for the determined poisoner. In Renaissance Europe, it was dubbed "inheritance powder" for the way it adjusted family fortunes and shaped the family trees of that continent's royal houses. Its ubiquity stemmed from its uncanny ability to mimic the symptoms of ordinary gastric ailments. Very few doctors—then or now—treating a patient convulsed by vomiting, cramps, dizziness and diarrhea would instinctively diagnose arsenical poisoning, and even if they did harbor suspicions, only a toxicology report could tell them for certain. (Until a London chemist named James Marsh developed his "arsenic mirror" in 1836, there was no way of telling conclusively if a human had ingested arsenic.) Besides being a wondrously efficient extinguisher of human life, arsenic is just as lethal on pests such as rats and ants.

If Terro Ant Killer *had* been introduced into the paramedics' diet, then it wouldn't have been the first time that this product had figured in the toxicology crime annals. In 1958 a glamorous thirty-three-year-old restaurateur from Macon, Georgia, named Anjette Lyles, was sentenced to the electric chair for feeding Terro to her nine-year-old daughter. (She almost certainly poisoned three other relatives as well.) She was later reprieved and remanded to the state mental hospital where she died in December 1977.

Grim-faced, the paramedics studied the bottle of Terro Ant Killer. Not one of them doubted that the contents of this innocuous looking bottle were responsible for their mystery ailment. To test this conviction, on October 19, 1984, they laid a trap for Swango. They purposely left a pitcher of freshly brewed unsweetened iced tea in the refreshment room at a time when they knew Swango would have unobserved access. When he was seen to leave the room hurriedly, then get in his car and roar off, the paramedics returned. One of them tasted the tea. It was sweet. This was the clincher. Because ants are attracted to anything sweet, the manufacturers of Terro had mixed the arsenic in a sucrose solution for maximum effectiveness. Carefully, the paramedics poured the iced tea into another container and sent it for chemical analysis. To no one's surprise the report came back positive—the iced tea had been spiked with arsenic.*

---

*Now, in the interest of greater public safety, the manufacturers of Terro Ant Killer use borax as the active ingredient, rather than arsenic.

When these findings, and details of the circumstances surrounding them, were passed to the Adams County Sheriff's Department, their reaction was swift. They obtained search warrants for Swango's apartment and also a storage unit he had rented. The combined haul uncovered an extraordinary cache of various chemicals, several bottles of ant killer, handwritten recipes for poisons, a scrapbook stuffed with newspaper cuttings of the 1982 Tylenol killings, castor beans—source of the deadly poison ricin—as well as an assortment of guns and knives. On October 26, 1984, Michael Swango was taken into custody and charged with poisoning six coworkers. Unfortunately, what no one realized at the time was that Swango and "clouds of suspicion" went hand in hand due mainly to the fact that wherever the smiling blond doctor went, he seemed to leave a trail of dead bodies in his wake.

His beginnings were mundane enough. Joseph Michael Swango—like his father he would never use his first name—was born on October 21, 1954, at Fort Lewis, just south of Tacoma, Washington. For most of his early childhood he was the classic "army brat," shuttling from one base to another, wherever Colonel J. Virgil Swango's military career took him. In 1967 the family finally settled in Quincy, Illinois, two hours north of St. Louis. Adolescence is never an easy time, and in Swango's early teens his father was posted overseas on the first of two tours of duty in Vietnam. Whatever effect this dislocation may have had on Swango's emotional development, it made no discernible impact on his studies. With a reported IQ in the 160s, he breezed through high school, easily conquering any subject, always obtaining the highest grade point average in the class. His real forte, though, was music. By his senior year he played the clarinet well enough to be made president of the school band. Honors and awards were heaped on his shoulders, so it came as no surprise when he graduated as valedictorian of the Class of '72, and was voted "most likely to succeed" by his classmates.

At home things weren't quite so idyllic. Raising four sons with an absent husband had taken its toll on Muriel Swango. And when Virgil finally came home from Vietnam for good, their marriage, always rocky, began to crumble. Neighbors became used to the sound of raised voices emanating from the pink bungalow late at night and took mental bets on how long the union would survive. The answer was "not very." Already a stranger to his family, Virgil now cut himself off from them completely, retreating into the alcoholic haze that would eventually kill him in 1982.

There is no evidence that Swango was ever really close to his father, although in later life he did develop a tendency to hype his father's Vietnam record somewhat. He had his clarinet and he had his studies and that seemed to be enough. Following graduation he won a full music scholarship to Millikin University in Decatur, Illinois, but after two semesters he quit and, to his mother's horror, announced that he was joining the Marines as a medic. Muriel freaked. Having already lost her husband to the military, the prospect of her favorite son following in his father's footsteps was almost too much for her to bear. The next two years of her life were thoroughly miserable as she fretted and pined over Michael's perceived rashness. Then, as suddenly as he had gone, Swango was back home with a brand new career path mapped out—he was going to be a doctor.

He laid the groundwork for this ambition at Quincy College, where once again he excelled academically, graduating in 1979 with honors and degrees in both chemistry and biology. From there he headed to the medical school at Southern Illinois University in Springfield. And it was here that the high school prodigy abruptly ran out of steam.

Perhaps it was because the academic temperature around him had suddenly risen by several degrees, or maybe the demons that would one day overtake him for good were just beginning to kick in, but for the first time in his life Swango struggled to keep up. He was trapped in an all too familiar vicious cycle: in order to pay his tuition fees, he needed to work, and the hours devoted to that task gouged deeply into his study time. To make some extra money—and in flagrant violation of school rules—he worked nights and weekends as an ambulance paramedic. The tab for this erratic lifestyle became payable at exam time. Then he would stay up all hours cramming frantically. And when cramming failed to do the trick, as his fellow students noted, he wasn't above a spot of blatant cheating.

Swango's exam-time deviousness might have slipped through the cracks had it not been for his all too obvious lack of interest in the "clinicals," the hands-on training that forms an integral part of the medical student's final stages. His attitude to patients nauseated his classmates. At best he was apathetic or sloppy; at worst he could be downright callous. Other students began calling him "Double-O Swango," jeering that he had a "license to kill." But it was no joking matter. Class tensions that had been simmering throughout Swango's tenure boiled over at the end of his final year when a delegation of students took their concerns to the teaching committee; they wanted him kicked out of school. The committee, after hearing both sides, decided to grant Swango a partial reprieve. Instead of expulsion, they opted to hold him back a year. It was a fudge that satisfied no one. The students felt the committee had shirked its responsibilities; Swango seethed because having to repeat his final year meant that dreams of a promised residency at the University of Iowa had now gone up in smoke.

Eventually, after considerable difficulty, he did graduate in obstetrics and gynecology, and in July 1983 he applied for a three-year neurosurgery residency at Ohio State University Hospitals. They accepted him but attached a rider: first, he had to complete a year-long internship in general surgery.

Swango struggled from the outset. Six months into his internship, a rash of low test scores brought a warning that his future acceptance into the neurosurgery program was teetering on a knife edge. "Straighten up or take a hike," was the message, and to show they meant business, his superiors placed him on probation. Swango was sailing perilously close to the wind. Soon, though, the ineptitude of Michael Swango was relegated to the backburner, as the hospital found itself having to cope with a new and far more dangerous problem—a wholly unprecedented surge in the number of code blue emergency calls.

The crisis peaked on February 6, 1984, when a student nurse named Carolyn Berry, on a routine ward check, was startled to see a young intern bend over an elderly patient, fiddle with the intravenous tube, then quickly dart from the room as if he didn't want to be seen. Just moments later, sixty-nine-year-old Rena Cooper grabbed hold of her bedrails and began shaking violently, gasping for breath. Berry called an immediate code blue, and the cardiac arrest team came running. During the course of what was, fortunately, a successful resuscitation, another nurse happened to see this same doctor sneaking out of a room four doors down. She, too, was struck by his furtive manner. Cautiously she decided to investigate. Inside the room, lying on a sink, was a syringe with a large needle—the kind used to penetrate plastic IV tubes. When the two nurses swapped stories, their misgivings grew. Rena Cooper, too, had no doubt that something very strange had happened. Her last memory, right before the sudden attack, was of a young doctor injecting some fluid into her IV tube.

That doctor was none other than Michael Swango.

The Cooper incident opened the floodgates. A rush of other nurses now came forward, all with disturbing stories about several deaths and near deaths that had happened in the preceding weeks. In each instance, Swango had been seen lurking close by, syringe in hand. Although it seemed too fantastic for words, several nurses were convinced that the young intern was deliberately killing the patients. One nurse added it up: there had been more code-blue alerts during the one month that Swango was on her ward than in the entire previous year.

Rather than involve the police—with the attendant publicity—the hospital decided to conduct an internal inquiry. They did a lousy job. Evidence, including syringes that the nurses had saved and some of the IV tubes, was either misplaced or lost. And nobody seemed to question the fact that, in separate interviews, Swango gave diametrically conflicting accounts of his whereabouts at the moments leading up to the Cooper code blue. One version had him admitting that he was in the patient's room; another placed him somewhere else entirely. After a week-long investigation, the inquiry was discreetly shut down. But the doubts had not been erased.

In March 1984, Swango received a letter from the hospital telling him that he would not be accepted into the neurosurgery residency program the following term. The details were necessarily vague, but OSU made one thing crystal clear—they didn't want Swango around.

Swango's parting shot at the institution that had fired him came three months later, right at the end of his internship. His fellow doctors were delighted with the bucket of Kentucky Fried Chicken and sodas that the smiling Swango produced and helped themselves. Inside an hour, all of them were heaving like sailboats in a hurricane. Some, scheduled to work in the operating room, ended up actually vomiting through their face masks. It never crossed anyone's mind that they might have been deliberately poisoned—until they heard what happened to the Quincy paramedics.

Swango's poisoning trial began on April 22, 1985. The case would be heard by Judge Dennis Cashman, without the benefit of a jury. Just about the only point at issue was whether the paramedics had actually ingested arsenic and this was proved by analyzing hair samples taken from each man. All showed abnormal levels of arsenic contamination. What Cashman heard from the paramedics and other witnesses convinced him that Swango was treating his victims "like his own little laboratory rats," first poisoning them and then studying their reactions. Cashman also suspected that the blatancy of Swango's crimes was deliberate, calculated to create the maximum publicity, ensuring that he would be caught and then placed in a position where his intellectual brilliance would win the day in court.

It didn't work out that way. After a two-week trial, Swango was convicted on six counts of aggravated battery. In one of the more prescient announcements to come from the bench in recent decades, Cashman told Swango, "It is obvious that you are a danger to this community and to any other place you may go." Hot on the heels of this verdict, Illinois immediately suspended Swango's medical license, while Ohio initiated proceedings to the same end.

At the penalty phase of the trial, held on August 23, Judge Cashman listened as Swango pleaded his case. "I am innocent of these charges," he declared. "In no way, shape or form, under no conceivable circumstances, am I now or could I ever be, a danger to any human being on the face of the earth." The prisoner went on to promise that, if given probation, he'd be "a productive member of society." Cashman wasn't impressed. "I accept your statement," he said. "But I don't accept it as true." He then jailed Swango for five years on each count. Just about the only surprise was that the sentences were concurrent: with time off for good behavior, Swango would be back on the streets after just a couple years.

As Swango was led away to begin his sentence, he did so in the knowledge that his home state of Illinois had revoked his medical license for good. Things looked blacker still in Ohio. There, it was rumored that the authorities were actively investigating Swango in the deaths of at least six Ohio State hospital patients under his care during 1983 and 1984. However, Franklin County prosecutors admitted that too much evidence had been lost to file charges. This did nothing to salvage Swango's medical license in Ohio, which was revoked. It looked as if Swango's medical days were over for good.

All his life Swango had been a masterful manipulator, and donning a prison uniform did nothing to dull that talent. Quite the contrary; he became something of a celebrity. In January 1986 this amiable solipsist gave an interview to ABC News's 20/20, in which he stated without any trace of irony, "I simply could not have done those things." All

his excuses were delivered with the open-faced disingenu-
ousness that had become Swango's trademark. This TV appearance did spark a brief flurry of publicity, but then the
disgraced former doctor became old news and faded from
public memory.

He resurfaced on August 21, 1987, when, after serving
just two years, he was released from the Centralia
Correctional Center. There were plenty of well-wishers on
hand. Even a member of the prosecution team that had put
Swango behind bars sounded upbeat. "He [Swango] is one
man who certainly has the intelligence and the ability to
make a positive contribution to society," said Chet Vahle,
former assistant state's attorney and now a circuit judge. "I
hope his problems are behind him." It was some hope.

Upon his release, Swango moved to Newport News,
Virginia and, calling himself David Adams, wangled a job
as an admissions officer at a medical vocational school and
placement agency. There, the strange duality in his personality deepened and widened; for despite being possessed of
immense personal charm, he always maintained his distance from other staff members. He wasn't standoffish, just
extraordinarily self-contained, set apart from everyone else
in the world. In May 1989 a coworker, curious to discover
the contents of the brown paper bag that accompanied
Adams everywhere, peeked inside and found it stuffed full
of newspaper clippings. All dealt with the poisoning trial
of someone called Michael Swango. Shortly thereafter,
three coworkers became violently sick with symptoms
eerily similar to those that struck down the Quincy paramedics. As the rumors began to circulate, an employee at
the agency passed on her suspicions to her ex-husband, a
police officer. He did some digging. When a check of criminal records revealed Swango's true identity, the police decided to search his house. If Swango was up to his old

tricks, this time it didn't show. Although officers turned his house upside down, they found nothing to connect him with any crime.

All this upheaval made Swango's position at the agency untenable and so he moved on. Not too far, though, just to a nearby laboratory, where he landed a job testing coal samples. Once again his highly vocal obsession with serial killers and violent crime made him a talking point among his fellow workers, most of whom began to experience the skin-crawling sense of unease that Swango generated wherever he went.

Time might have closed many doors for Swango, but it had done nothing to dilute his determination to pursue some kind of medically related work. He enrolled in a Hampton, Virginia, paramedic training program, and graduated in December 1990, somehow circumventing a state prohibition against convicted felons becoming emergency medical technicians. Armed with this qualification, Swango took a part-time paramedic's job with Medical Transport Inc. in Suffolk, Virginia. During the course of his day-to-day duties he quite naturally visited several of the local medical facilities, and in November 1991 he happened to enter Sentara Hampton General Hospital. The on-duty nurse could scarcely believe her eyes. She recognized Swango from his time at Ohio and immediately alerted hospital officials. They in turn contacted the Ohio State Medical Board, who divulged full details of Swango's conviction and the suspicious events at Ohio State University Hospitals.

When this information eventually filtered through to the Virginia state EMT licensing board, Swango was called in and asked to explain himself. He oozed his customary charm and promised to deliver the paperwork they requested. The fact that the documents were not forthcoming was neither here nor there, because in March 1992 Swango had another job offer on the table—he was going to be a doctor again.

Ever since 1990, Swango had been firing off applications to medical schools right across America. He'd tried West Virginia, Virginia, Washington, DC, and North Dakota, and each time revelations about his troubled past came back to haunt him. Swango had his explanation ready. Yes, he'd served time, but that was the result of a barroom brawl in his younger and wilder youth. Moreover, he brandished documentation—a docket sheet from the Illinois court and a "release fact sheet" from the Illinois Department of Correction—to back up his claims (both documents were later found to be forgeries). When queried over his name change, he sorrowfully explained that an undisclosed family problem had forced him to use an alias. Swango's barefaced lies usually stood up for as long as it took someone on the interviewing board to reach for the telephone. In short order, all the medical schools turned him down flat. Except the University of South Dakota at Sioux Falls.

At that time in South Dakota, a felony conviction was no automatic bar to holding a medical license; it all depended on the seriousness of the charge. University officials considered Swango's carefully rehearsed story of the barroom brawl, and decided that he merited a second chance. He was offered a family practice residency beginning July 1992. But Nemesis was always peeking over his shoulder.

Just five months into his training, on November 28, a local cable channel rebroadcast an edited version of his *20/20* interview. When the faculty members at USD saw the program, jaws dropped and pulses began racing. Moves were immediately put in place to expel Swango. In typical fashion, Swango made no attempt to shun the local media, instead he went into full-on "victim mode," insisting that he had been utterly transparent about his background when interviewed. It was scarcely his fault, he said, if the panel then chose to mislead the university board. Full marks for chutzpah, maybe, but all the bluster and bombast in the world couldn't get him out of this mess. The upshot was that he'd been blacklisted by yet another state, and, in January 1993, when his appeal process expired, he limped back to Newport News with his tail very much between his legs.

It didn't take him long to bounce back onto his feet. The following April found him at Stony Brook Veterans Hospital in Long Island, New York, where he caught a sympathetic ear on the interviewing board as he rehashed that careworn saga of the barroom indiscretion. Swango's earnest contrition, bolstered by his avowed determination to seek a new start, won the day. Out of 190 applicants for a place on the four-year psychiatric medicine residency program, he was one of only a dozen to gain a place. So powerful had been his presentation that the hospital decided not to bother checking out his biographical details.

No sooner had Swango begun training at the VA Hospital in Northport in July 1993, than a strange kind of malaise began creeping through the wards. Some patients died quite unexpectedly; others saw their symptoms mysteriously worsen and change. One of the latter was Barron Harris, a sixty-year-old Vietnam veteran from Holbrook, New York. On October 2, he was admitted to the hospital suffering from pneumonia, an illness that was serious but not considered life threatening. And then he received a visit from Michael Swango. After ingesting some pills, Harris abruptly lapsed into a coma. It was a similar story with another pneumonia patient, Andrew Woods. He, too, suffered seizures after swallowing some of Swango's medication.

An internal investigation into these and all the other disturbing incidents at Stony Brook over that summer isolated one common factor—Michael Swango. On October 13, he was fired. Shortly thereafter the staff member responsible for hiring Swango resigned, admitting he had made "a terrible mistake" in not checking the applicant's background.

Once again Swango was hot news. And yet, oddly enough, for once this most media-friendly of medics was nowhere to be found. The man branded by his former boss at Stony Brook as a "charming, pathological liar," had seemingly disappeared from the face of the earth.

In his wake he left further tragedy. In the early hours of November 8, Barron Harris, who had never regained consciousness from the coma, died. His wife immediately announced her intention of suing the hospital. Woods, too, decided to go to the law.

The avalanche of negative publicity that attended Swango's latest imbroglio came as no surprise to Illinois Circuit Judge Dennis Cashman, the jurist who had sentenced Swango to prison for the Quincy poisonings. He had tracked each new revelation with a mixture of revulsion and anger, and he wasn't reticent about pointing the finger of blame. In a string of interviews, he lambasted the medical community, charging them with "supreme arrogance," for the way they had believed Swango just because he was a doctor, as though a physician's word was somehow sacrosanct. Shamefaced agreement with this verdict came from Dr. Robert Talley, dean of the medical school at the University of South Dakota. "In retrospect," he said, "one would have to say that's the case."

The cleanup campaign, however belated, now swung into purposeful action. On October 25, 1995, the dean of the School of Medicine at Stony Brook circulated a letter to 125 medical schools and 1,500 teaching hospitals across America detailing Swango's record, warning that he was likely to use aliases and any other necessary subterfuge to gain admittance to their programs.

With the lawsuits piling up, and the police and the Justice Department trying to figure out what, if anything, Swango could be charged with, the center of all this activity was proving to be maddeningly elusive. Eventually he was tracked down to a friend's house near Atlanta and placed under discreet surveillance. This surveillance took on a renewed urgency when it was learned that Swango had obtained a job at a water treatment facility that fed into Atlanta's water supply. The prospect was too appalling to contemplate, but even before the authorities could warn the water company, Swango left.

In October 1994, the long-anticipated arrest warrant, charging Swango with having lied on his application to join the federally funded VA hospital at Stony Brook, finally materialized. But by then it was too late: Swango had vanished once again.

And when he surfaced, the wannabe doctor was half a world away.

Western-trained physicians are welcomed with open arms in Africa, and the agency that leafed through Swango's application was genuinely excited. His resume was as impressive as it was fanciful, complete with forged references and glowing commendations from medical establishments across the United States, and all imbued with Swango's stated desire to treat some of the most disadvantaged people on earth. The agency had no difficulty finding Swango a position.

Mnene is a flyspeck on the map of south-central

Zimbabwe. It lies about 120 miles southeast of Bulawayo, deep in the bush, and its grazing grounds are home to two hundred thousand people, most of whom scratch a meager living from the animals they tend. Just three tiny medical facilities serve this region and it was to one of these, Mnene Mission Hospital, with its bungalows and verandas, that "Doctor Mike" was sent.

For most of the locals, it was as if a benevolent alien had dropped in from another planet. Handsome, smiling Doctor Mike bowled everyone over with his eye-catching blend of good looks and bottomless charm. The mission director, Dr. Christopher Zshiri, might have privately speculated why a forty-year-old American doctor with such glowing qualifications and no previous history of altruism would suddenly decide to forgo a huge salary in his homeland to practice in such an out-of-the-way spot, but like everyone else at Mnene, he was just grateful to have Swango on board, and so he kept his concerns to himself.

Over the first few weeks Zshiri monitored Swango's work from a discreet distance, and what he saw disturbed him. For someone whose credentials read like an Ivy League graduation parade, the newcomer seemed remarkably naive when it came to basic medical care. In Mnene it wasn't cutting edge medicine that the locals needed, but solid no-nonsense attention to routine childbirths, wounds, cysts, broken limbs, that kind of thing, and when it came to these, Swango didn't have a clue. Zshiri took the newcomer to one side and it was agreed that he should take a five-month internship at Mpilo Hospital in Bulawayo to familiarize himself with the fundamentals of doctoring the local populace. When Swango returned to Mnene in May 1995, his technique had improved out of all recognition, but his attitude had soured. Sloppy timekeeping and unauthorized vacations were just two of his flaws, all exacerbated by an increasingly supercilious attitude he adopted toward the nuns who acted as nurses at the mission. But worse was to come.

The first person to die was Rhoda Mahlamvana. She entered Mnene Mission Hospital suffering from burns received in an accident and appeared to be responding well to treatment. Until Doctor Mike took over her case. On May 24, she died suddenly. Swango seemed as puzzled as anyone else by her unexpected demise.

A few weeks later, Katazo Shava also seemed well on the road to recovery after a leg operation and was joking with friends when Swango suddenly appeared and shooed everyone from the room. Moments later, an unearthly scream rang out. When the friends ran back they found Shava trembling violently, crying that the doctor had injected him with something. Shava's agony lasted into the afternoon, when he died. Swango signed the death certificate himself, writing in "heart failure."

That same day, Philimon Chipoko underwent an operation to amputate his foot. It was a routine operation and there were no complications, and yet in the early hours of the next morning, June 27, Chipoko was found dead. His wife, Yeudzirai, confided to the nurses that she had seen Swango come in around 11 PM and bend over her husband to carry out some procedure. Again it was Swango's signature on the death certificate, "heart failure."

So many unaccountable deaths in such close proximity to each other inevitably set tongues wagging, and most of the gossip concerned Doctor Mike. In time a schism opened up in the nursing staff, with one camp decidedly anti-Swango, the other strongly supportive of the volunteer from America.

Following this outbreak of tragedies there was a lull.

The next suspicious death to hit Mnene came on July 17, when Edith Ngwenya, a nursing aide who had been one of Swango's staunchest defenders, died around 11:25 AM. She was pronounced dead by Swango, who completed the death certificate and listed the cause of death as pneumonia.

Two days later it was Margaret Zhou's turn. She had undergone a routine operation to right the effects of an incomplete abortion. Again there had been no difficulties, and yet she suddenly died. This string of disasters had to be stopped, the nuns decided. A deputation went to Zshiri and demanded that something be done about Swango.

For the first time, Zshiri heard about irregularities in Swango's method of treatment, especially his insistence on personally administering injections to all his patients. Ordinarily this was a job performed by nurses, and it was certainly odd that Swango would delegate this task to himself. Two patients, who had survived surprise injections from Swango and were still receiving treatment in hospital, now told Zshiri their stories.

On May 14, a man in his mid-fifties, Keneas Mzezewa, had been fast asleep at night when he felt a strange pricking sensation in his arm. As he awoke he saw Swango hovering over him. Then the doctor did something most peculiar—he waved good-bye and left. A short time later, Mzezewa felt like he was on fire, unable to move his limbs, gasping for breath. Summoning one superhuman last effort he managed a single scream. The nurses came running. Almost miraculously they revived the stricken man, then listened to his terrified story. Swango dismissed Mzezewa's complaints as hallucinatory ravings, and bitterly denied having administered any injection. But what the outwardly indignant Swango failed to appreciate was that the nurses had already found part of a syringe by the patient's bed.

Two months later, and Virginia Sibanda's expected normal childbirth turned out to be anything but when Swango barged his way into the delivery room and took charge. While the nurses were otherwise distracted, Sibanda said, Swango produced a syringe from inside his white coat and plunged it into her. Like Mzezewa, she felt the full impact of the injection almost right away. An excruciating pain wracked her whole body. Her cries for help did not go unheeded and the nurses were able to save both mother and child.

When confronted about this incident, Swango fell back on his threadbare excuse of "delusions" on the part of the patient. But Zshiri had heard enough. He contacted the police and they obtained a search warrant for the small cottage that Swango called home.

Inside, they found a ramshackle collection of death-dealing drugs, syringes and dozens of open ampoules and bottles. Most ominous of all was the vial of potassium chloride, the literally heart-stopping agent used in capital punishment by lethal injection. As there was no reason for Swango to have any of these drugs in his personal possession, he was suspended immediately.

Swango cried foul, and hired a lawyer to pursue a civil suit against the hospital. To gain some breathing space, he retreated to the relative safety of Bulawayo, where he somehow managed to finagle a job at Mpilo Hospital. When Zshiri found out he was mortified and immediately contacted Mpilo. They listened to Zshiri's warning—and did absolutely nothing. How much their decision was influenced by Swango's offer to work for nothing except his accommodation must remain a matter for conjecture.

What made things doubly disturbing was the fact that

Swango's lodgings were immediately adjacent to the hospital wards, and this meant he could come and go at any time of the day or night without being seen. Within days patients began dying. Because records were not kept so meticulously as at Mnene, the number of suspicious Mpilo deaths can only be estimated. The figure most often mentioned is fifteen. All were patients unfortunate enough to come into close contact with Doctor Mike, and all died without any prior warning.

With the Mpilo body count rising almost daily, communications were winging their way around the globe demanding details of Michael Swango's background. Once the full picture became clear, the Ministry of Health in Harare contacted Mpilo and ordered them to get rid of Swango and banish him from the hospital premises. Swango took refuge with a woman friend in Malindela, a city in Matabeleland North Province. Throughout his stay, he remained in constant telephone contact with his lawyer, and heard that state prosecutors were building a strong case. In August 1996, he was summoned to appear at a hearing to decide his future. But Swango didn't show.

At some time around August 14, he hopped a Blue Arrow bus and fled northward into the neighboring state of Zambia. (He hadn't even bothered to collect the $35,000 damages he had been awarded in a hospital lawsuit.) One thing he hadn't abandoned, though, was his ineradicable charisma; it landed him a job straight away, working as a doctor at the University Teaching Hospital in Lusaka, Zambia. The respite was only temporary, however. It might have been a different country, but Swango couldn't leave his past behind. It was stalking him like a lion hunter.

In November 1996, news finally reached officials at the Lusaka hospital about the deaths in Zimbabwe, and

Swango was shown the door. The next stop on his African safari was Namibia in the southwest of the continent. In March 1997, using a PO box in Windhoek, he sent his resume to an agency that hired doctors in Saudi Arabia. Judging from the fanciful answers on the application form, his powers of invention were undiminished. Certainly the agency was impressed and in May they offered Swango a position at a hospital in Dhahran, the desert enclave specifically built to house employees of the Aramco oil company and their families. It sounded like the dream post, well paid, first-rate facilities, fabulous weather, beautiful accommodation, and—most reassuringly of all—thousands of miles away from anyone who knew him.

There was only one drawback: he needed a visa. And that visa had to be obtained in Swango's country of birth. Despite his repeated attempts to have the visa issued in Africa, the Saudi authorities would not budge. All his life Swango had been a risk-taker, now he decided to take the biggest gamble of all. He would fly back to the US and get the required visa.

On June 27, 1997, Swango landed at Chicago's O'Hare Airport. The stopover was intended to be brief, just pick up the visa and catch another plane to Saudi Arabia. But it didn't turn out that way. The FBI computers that check all passport numbers against flight arrivals and departures had flagged Swango as a wanted fugitive. That old warrant about lying on his application to Stony Brook was still valid. Michael Swango's running days were over for good.

He was taken into custody and arraigned on charges of fraud. Initially he attempted to bluster and to smooth talk his way out of trouble, but gradually as the hopelessness of his situation became apparent, he decided to deal. Lurking in the back of his mind was the knowledge that he was getting off lightly. At a hearing held on July 12, 1998, Swango pleaded guilty to the fraud charges and was sentenced to forty-two months. The judge ordered that, throughout his incarceration, Swango should be denied access to any duty that involved the preparation or delivery of food. With time off for good behavior—and Swango had always been a model prisoner—he could expect to be out after two years.

This terrifying prospect galvanized law enforcement minds on two continents. As the release deadline drew near, and the race heated up to find the definitive evidence that would prove Swango a heartless murderer, FBI agents went back through Swango's records and isolated that string of suspicious deaths during his time at Stony Brook VA hospital. They zeroed in on three incidents.

The first of these concerned George Siano, a construction worker from Shirley, New York, who died shortly after Swango started at the hospital. For two weeks Swango had been treating Siano, aged seventy, for cancer. Siano's case notes, in Swango's own hand, ended on July 26, 1993, with the ominous conclusion "no chance of recovery." Swango was writing no more than the truth. Seven years later, after Siano's body had been exhumed, toxicologists were able to confirm the presence of unauthorized drugs.

The second victim, Aldo Serini, was a sixty-two-year-old veteran of the Korean War who had suffered a nervous breakdown. He had been a psychiatric patient at Northport for more than twenty years, and on September 23, 1993, he suddenly began to suffer problems with his breathing. Part of his treatment included being hooked up to an IV line. While a puzzled nurse looked on, Swango, with a conjurer's flourish, suddenly produced a syringe from inside his lab coat. Thinking that he intended to flush Serini's IV with a saline solution, the nurse remained quiet as Swango injected the contents of the syringe into the plastic tube. What happened next was really bizarre. Ordinarily, in a busy hospital a doctor moved on after treating a patient. But not Swango. For two hours he remained in Serini's room, sometimes sitting on the radiator, sometimes bending over the patient, but all the while watching intently until the man eventually drifted into unconsciousness. The last action Swango performed for Serini was to forge a DNR form—"Do Not Resuscitate"—making it appear as if the form had been signed by a family member. Sure enough, Serini died.

Thomas Sammarco had also been attending Northport hospital for twenty years, after paralyzing his legs in a fall. In all that time Sammarco had borne his infirmity with uplifting cheerfulness that warmed everyone who knew him. But in 1993 all that changed. This time he had gone into hospital for elective open heart surgery. The procedure had been a success and yet Sammarco's mood seemed, unaccountably, to change for the worse. He began to hallucinate, insistent that someone was trying to kill him. He raved about "a man with a medical cart who waved as he passed him in the night." The family was told that seventy-three-year-old Sammarco was suffering from mental confusion. And then, on October 3, 1993, Sammarco abruptly lapsed into a coma. That night, as he lay in intensive care, his daughter, Carol Fischer, waited anxiously at his bedside. As if this ordeal were not trying enough, throughout she was pestered by the doctor on duty to sign a DNR, even though she had already completed this grim formality with another physician. Swango, eager to cover his tracks as thoroughly as possible, oozed his customary charm. The other doctor, he explained condescendingly, was very young and underqualified for such a responsibility. Worn down by Swango's persistence, Carol duly signed a second form. The next day her father was dead.

These three deaths, the FBI decided, represented the

government's best chances of convincing a jury that Michael Swango was a serial killer. In early 2000, family members gave permission for exhumations to be conducted on all three bodies. Test results showed that all three men had been poisoned by various drugs that included the powerful muscle relaxants succinylcholine and epinephrine.

The suspense came right down to the wire. Just four days before Swango was scheduled for release, agents charged him with triple murder. Ever since college, the man from Quincy had dealt himself into the highest stakes poker game around—killing humans and avoiding capture. Now, though, the federal government had raised the ante. Facing the certainty of a death sentence if convicted, Swango was in no mood to bluff. On September 6, 2000, looking thin and unsmiling, he appeared in court, and each time Judge Jacob Mishler asked Swango how he pleaded to murder, he received the impassive answer: "Guilty, your honor." In what came as a shock to almost everyone present, Swango also admitted to another killing, one he had committed a decade before his VA hospital murder spree.

Cynthia McGee, a nineteen-year-old gymnast at the University of Illinois, had been cycling by the campus at Urbana on November 4, 1983, when she was struck by a speeding Corvette. Rushed to the hospital in Champaign, Cynthia recovered enough to be transferred to a hospital nearer her home in Ohio. For the final stage of her treatment, she was in OSU Hospital at Columbia. Despite being well on the way to what was later called a "storybook recovery," on January 15, 1984, she died. Following her death, the teenage driver of the Corvette, Scott Bone, was convicted of reckless homicide, and sentenced to thirty months' probation and one thousand hours of community service. He also lost his license for several years.

Tragically for everyone concerned, at the same time that Cynthia was bedridden at OSU Hospital, Michael Swango was prowling the wards on his internship. And on January 14, 1984, he injected McGee with a lethal dose of potassium.*

Because the murder of Cynthia McGee was not a federal offense, it was not listed on the indictment against Swango. It made little difference to the outcome. He was sentenced to three life terms with no possibility of parole. At the time of writing, Swango is incarcerated at the Administrative Maximum Facility at Florence, Colorado. He will remain behind bars for the rest of his life.

Only Michael Swango knows exactly how many people he killed. Estimates range from thirty-five to sixty, mostly African, although it should be noted that no publicly available evidence exists to justify these numbers. What is undeniable is his place among the most prolific serial killers of all time. As always in cases like this, the baffled onlooker wants to know "Why?" In all probability, like his unconscious mentor, Dr. Harold Shipman, Swango "found the drama of taking life to his taste." Certainly this seems borne out by scribblings contained in a notebook confiscated from Swango at the time of his arrest at O'Hare Airport. They reveal his utter addiction to the habit of killing. In his spidery writing, he had dutifully copied passages from various novels that he felt could inform his murderous activities. One such extract slavered over the "sweet, husky, close smell of an indoor homicide." Another read: "When I kill someone, it's because I want to.

---

*On July 12, 2001, Bone had his conviction overturned and his record cleared.

It's the only way I have of reminding myself that I'm still alive."

So there we have it, the chilling realization that, in order for Dr. Michael Swango to experience a few fleeting moments of feeling fully "alive," untold numbers of families have been forced to suffer the permanent wrench of death.

6. THE SINS OF THE FATHER

At times the bond between doctor and patient borders on the supernatural. Logic plays no part in it; loyalty is all. Such was the case with Dr. John Dale Cavaness. He was a drunk, a bully, a fraud and a lecher, but folks in the scrubby rural South Illinois town of Harrisburg worshipped him. Even after he was arraigned on the kind of murder charge that most find hard to imagine, let alone countenance, people stuck by him. The words of one patient said it all: "Well, even if he did do it, I hope and pray that they can't prove it." Over the years Cavaness had looked after them and now it was time for the town to rally behind him. Many of them had already done so for years, even to the point of sitting back and turning a blind eye while Dr. Dale Cavaness remorselessly killed off his own sons, one by one.

The object of all this devotion was born on October 15, 1925, in Eldorado, Illinois. Whoever named the town had some sense of humor; Eldorado didn't have too much in the way of gold, just coal. For a few decades the ugly strip mines lined local pockets but, during the Depression, Eldorado went the way of countless midwestern towns. The mines closed down and people moved away, either northwest to St. Louis or else the longer trip to Chicago. Those who stayed just got on with life as best they could. The pickings were lean. Poverty brought with it a disregard for outside rules and, especially, outside interference. More often than not arguments in Eldorado were still settled with fists and bullets. Feuds ran deep and long, and nobody liked whiners; if you had a problem, then you were expected to fix it on your own account and not go snivelling to some nosy lawman. In Eldorado that was the manly thing to do.

Given this kind of background, it was hardly surprising that Cavaness grew up the way he did. His mother, a preachy woman, big on the Bible, made him study the violin; his father made him fight. Gradually the fighting won. Cavaness thrived on brawling. And it was always the big kids he took on. He liked nothing better than punching it out with someone who outweighed him by several pounds or else towered over him. At first he might take a pounding, but Dale Cavaness would never give in and, ultimately, he would have them on the ground, smashing his fists into their faces until they pleaded with him to stop.

Almost uniquely in Eldorado the Cavaness family escaped the grinding deprivation of the Depression. Peck Cavaness had a job as brakeman on the railroad and kept it; he also owned a car. Younger than most, Dale Cavaness knew what it was to travel. Even if the horizons were somewhat limited, just the surrounding towns mostly, the experience still nurtured his ego and convinced him that he was a cut above the other boys at school. His mother kept him in good clothes and persisted with her dreams of her son playing the violin. Dale did little to accommodate her.

At Eldorado High School he became a fitness fanatic. He ran, pumped iron, worked out, eager to pack as much muscle as possible on his 5'7" frame. Despite his best efforts, he never weighed more than 150 lbs, but on the football gridiron his fiery competitiveness more than compensated for any lack of bulk. There was something maniacal about the way Dale Cavaness played football, almost as if he wanted to get hurt, just to show everyone how tough he was.

To his mother's relief this determination also spilled over into the classroom; learning was never a chore, rather something to be done insouciantly. But, as his academic and physical prowess increased, so did his cruelty. Always a practical joker, the gags now took on a meaner, more sadistic edge. One girl told how Dale asked to see her new watch, then deliberately dropped and crushed it beneath his foot. He ran off, hooting with laughter. Decades later she was one of the few unsurprised by the way Dale Cavaness turned out; she'd seen through the hail-fellow-well-met veneer and found a devil lurking.

While still in his teens, Cavaness decided on a career in medicine. All around him he could see the effects of poverty, neglect and malnutrition. Southern Illinois at this time was dirt poor. Whole families missed out on medical attention, usually because they couldn't afford it. This was a real chance to make a real difference in the community. Not that Cavaness was motivated by altruism alone. He also saw the way these people looked up to doctors. If he became a physician he would command that kind of respect; and respect was the one thing that Dale Cavaness craved, that and money.

All through high school he had been going out with Helen Jean Pearce, daughter of a local doctor. What started out as puppy love slowly grew into something more serious. For their part, Helen's parents were pleased at the match; Dale looked to be a lad with a future. Dr. Pearce encouraged him in his ambition, hinting that when Dale finished medical school there might be a place for him at the new hospital Pearce intended building.

But all that had to be put on hold; there was a war going on. Cavaness served two years in the navy, seeing duty in the Pacific. On his return to the States he and Helen wasted no time in getting married, much to the chagrin of Dale's mother. She resented Helen Jean, hated the way her own power over Dale was diminished. The relationship between Dale and his mother had always been peculiar. As an only child he'd been spoiled, of course, but Noma Cavaness took maternal devotion to another level, one which Dale loathed. He never missed a chance to publicly curse her, spitting that he wished she were dead.

Despite Noma's worst efforts, the young couple's marriage got off to a good start. Cavaness entered college on the GI bill and did well. He was known as the cocky student who could always back up his boasts. He breezed through the curriculum, received his BS and, in May 1947, began attending medical school in St. Louis.

Three years later came stunning news—Dale and Helen split up. The rift caught everyone unaware. There had been no hint of trouble, but Helen was quietly adamant; she didn't want to talk about it and she wanted to get out. Cavaness was less reticent. He told anyone who would listen that Helen had been cheating on him with his best friend. Sympathy came from all quarters. One of the most understanding was Marian Newberry, a close friend of Helen's. After the divorce she and Cavaness began dating regularly.

When Cavaness went to Baltimore to serve his internship, Marian took a job as an airline stewardess with the object of saving as much money as possible for their forth-coming marriage. They returned to St. Louis and tied the knot in October 1952. Because Cavaness had excelled ac-ademically, Marian took it for granted that he would aim for a top job on the East Coast. At the very least she thought he would do no worse than a big midwestern city. But in September 1954 Cavaness abruptly announced that they were moving to McLeansboro in Southern Illinois, just a few miles north of Eldorado. The country boy was going back home.

Cavaness had lined up a job at the Hamilton Memorial Hospital where hard work gained him a fine reputation and countless adoring patients. Socially, too, he and Marian were in great demand. Dale Cavaness was finally picking up the kind of respect he thought he deserved. But he had begun drinking heavily, and his temper when drunk was vi-cious. During one wedding anniversary he and Marian stayed at home to celebrate. The evening was fine until Marian tipsily giggled that she couldn't see herself spend-ing the rest of her life in McLeansboro. Cavaness didn't say a word, just punched her in the mouth. Next morning he claimed not to be able to remember the incident and it was never mentioned again.

That August they had their first son, Mark. Cavaness paid scant attention to the child; that was Marian's job, he was too busy with his practice. But, just as he seemed set for a really solid career, opportunity came knocking. Dr. Pearce, father of his ex-wife, offered him a position at the family hospital in Eldorado. Marian was shattered when Cavaness broke the news that they were moving back to his hometown. McLeansboro was bad enough; Eldorado would be impossible.

In 1955 they made the move. Dr. Pearce welcomed his

ex-son-in-law back with open arms. There was no animosity whatsoever; both he and his wife blamed their daughter for the marital break-up. Pearce saw Cavaness, with his fancy qualifications and up-to-the-minute methods of treatment, as a giant-size addition to the family hospital.

Cavaness quickly set about proving him right. He had a way of communicating with his patients, explaining their ailments, that built their confidence and made them look up to him. Another strong point in his favor was his seeming indifference about payment for services. Often he continued to treat people who owed him a great deal. More than anything else it was this trait that endeared Cavaness to his patients and explained their later loyalty. These folks would go to hell and back for Dr. Dale. However, unbeknownst to his legions of admirers, Cavaness always got paid one way or another, either falsifying insurance claims or else bending the workman's compensation laws. Later, when it became common knowledge, his patients would just shrug. In their eyes Cavaness was some kind of medical Robin Hood, robbing the insurance companies so that poor people could get treatment. They couldn't see much wrong with that at all.

They didn't even mind his warped humor, or those savage practical jokes. His favorite was to switch X-rays, then point out some ailment on the negative and tell people they were far sicker than they really were. One time he told a hapless woman that she was expecting twins. Only after she had gone out and bought a double stroller and duplicate sets of baby clothes did he own up and admit that the X-ray was of someone else. And still the patients laughed.

But things weren't so jovial at home. Noma Cavaness just couldn't keep her nose out of Dale's business, forever chiding Marian about the way she was raising Mark. Whenever Cavaness found out he would erupt. And each time he did, he always ended the same way, drinking himself into a fury, screaming how much he hated his mother, wishing that she were dead.

Marian had the patience of Job. All she wanted was a quiet, comfortable life. She got neither. Cavaness was never the kind to do anything by halves. If he was in a restaurant, he always had to be the life of the party. In bars he drank himself stupid and didn't consider the night over until he had picked a fight with someone. Afterward he would climb into his car and try to drive home. Oddly enough, the more folks in Eldorado learned about Cavaness the more they loved him. He hadn't got high and mighty on them; deep down he was just a good ole boy. He liked his drink and he liked his guns; automatics, rifles, shotguns, revolvers, pistols, anything. Eventually his home resembled a National Guard armory, with eighty-eight different firearms.

As the years passed Marian wearied of trying to change her husband. Optimistically she wondered if having a bigger family might calm him down. Baby Kevin came along in 1956. The new addition hardly affected Cavaness at all. The only time he ever paid any attention to his boys was to punish them. Once he deliberately locked Kevin in a darkened cupboard, went away and left him, then shouted at him for crying. That was the one trait he fought to instill in his boys: you had to be tough, any sign of emotion was an admission of weakness. He beat his kids till they cried, then beat them again for crying. If they lost a scrap at school and he got to hear about it, that meant another leathering.

And then there was the humiliation. One Christmas Kevin had asked for a special bike. On Christmas morning he came rushing down and found the bike beneath the tree. Ecstatic, he ran over to the bike, then saw the card that said

"Mark" pinned to it. He was crushed—Mark had never mentioned anything about wanting a bike. Cavaness sneered that Kevin shouldn't expect to get something just by whining about it. Later that day, after a row with Marian, Cavaness owned up; the bike had been for Kevin all along. He just wanted to teach his son a lesson, even on Christmas Day. Marian dissolved into tears, unable to believe any father could be so heartless.

Despite the money he made—and it was never less than six figures—Cavaness always yearned for more. Dreams of a vast empire led him to purchase several parcels of land, including two farms, and, being Dale Cavaness, of course he knew better than anyone else how to raise cattle. It was a matter of breeding, he told friends; with his knowledge of medicine he was going to combine the latest modern technology with traditional farming techniques and raise the biggest cattle in the world.

Even here his temper got the better of him. Out at the farm one day to supervise things, Cavaness became apoplectic when a prize bull refused to enter a trailer. Drunk and purple from rage, he rushed to his car and grabbed a .357 Magnum. With onlookers gaping in disbelief, Cavaness shot the $10,000 bull square in the eye. Pretty soon the story was added to the local legend of Dr. Dale. He did the damndest things sometimes!

The birth of his third son, Sean, in 1962, spurred Cavaness to even greater rages. His temper, always short, now operated on a hair trigger as he thrashed the boys unmercifully. Maybe if he had remained childless Dale Cavaness would have been different. Maybe not. Marian also came in for some brutal beatings. After one particularly savage attack Cavaness panted to his boys that he had just tried to kill their mother.

It was about this time that Marian caught Cavaness in

bed with another woman, her first intimation that he had ever been unfaithful. Sadly, it would not be the last. Doubling Marian's grief was the fact that she was pregnant again. Cavaness waited till she was six months gone before icily declaring that he wanted nothing more to do with her. They would continue to live together in the same house, but he would damn well come and go as he pleased and, if she didn't like it, then she knew what she could do. Choking back the tears, Marian nodded mute assent.

After the birth of yet another son, Patrick, Cavaness's violent abuse of Marian assumed ever more terrifying levels. Inevitably they separated, the only surprise being that it was Cavaness who left. At first he paid the bills but then his checks began to bounce. Marian, desperate for grocery money, went to see him. Cavaness looked her straight in the face and announced that he was broke.

He wasn't lying. All his get-rich-quick schemes had gone up in smoke. He was making plenty from his practice but the cattle rearing and catfish-farming businesses, designed to make him the richest man in Eldorado, were eating him alive. In desperation he plunged into the stock market, only to suffer the sickening sensation of watching his stock nosedive. Brokers badgered him daily, demanding more cash. For all his supposed cleverness, Dale Cavaness was clueless when it came to money. He needed someone to straighten him out financially, a first-rate bookkeeper.

Eddie Miller was just that, and, he soon put Cavaness's finances back in order. He paid the bills on time, collected overdue accounts, and always made sure that Marian and the boys were taken care of. Had Cavaness left everything in Miller's hands he might have survived, but that wasn't his style. He refused to accept that anyone could do anything better than himself, with the result that, in no time flat, Cavaness undid all the good that Miller had done, spending money faster than it came in. Miller's complaints were brushed off savagely. Like almost everyone in Eldorado he had idolized Cavaness, now a suspicion flickered deep within him that all was not well with this man. Maybe it was the booze? Cavaness was never without a drink. Even in his car he always kept a flask. He drove drunk and frequently worked that way as well. Those on the hospital staff aware of his habit refused to speak out against him. In large part Cavaness bought their silence by doling out methedrine and other amphetamines as though they were candy, to nurses, to clerks, to anyone who worked with him, until several of his employees found themselves hopelessly hooked.

Another of Miller's duties was buying presents for the harem of women that Cavaness maintained. Now that he was estranged his philandering reached epidemic proportions. All the affairs were of the "hump 'em, dump 'em" variety—quick conquests accompanied by lavish gifts, then abrupt dismissal. Invariably the onus for getting rid of the discards also fell on Miller. He hated the task, but did it anyway, out of love and respect for Dr. Dale. But by late 1968 Miller could take no more and gave in his notice.

Following his departure Marian's child-support checks resumed their bouncing ways. She pleaded with Cavaness for more money. He told her to get a job, stop leeching off him, then he coolly handed over a bagful of dirty laundry for her to wash. Swallowing her pride, Marian did his washing, fearful that, if she refused, Cavaness would cut off all semblance of financial assistance.

Just when it seemed that her life couldn't get any worse, on the afternoon of February 17, 1970 Marian's house burned down. She lost everything. The insurance company settled Cavaness's claim for $100,000 and Marian expected him to have the house rebuilt, but he seemed in no hurry. She and the boys had to live in a motel, penniless, making do with clothes borrowed from friends, none of whom could understand how a wealthy doctor's wife could find herself in such dire straits.

Marian bore her misery stoically and continued prodding her husband to take care of his family. Eventually Cavaness bought two trailers, one new, the other used. He placed them at the edge of town, telling Marian that they would have to do for now.

This was the final straw for Cavaness's parents. For years they had tolerated their son's excesses but no longer. When his father confronted him about the shabby way he was treating his family, Cavaness first told him to go to hell, then attempted to run him down in his car.

One year after the fire Cavaness had still made no effort to rebuild the house. Marian, assuming that he had blown the money, made preparations to move. But before she could, fate finally caught up with Cavaness.

He had been driving drunk again. There was nothing unusual about this; Cavaness was always ending up in some ditch or other, but this time his pickup had hit another car head-on late at night. The oncoming car was demolished, killing the driver and his ten-month-old daughter outright, critically injuring the mother. In Cavaness's truck police found an almost empty bottle of Scotch and the omnipresent .357 Magnum. Cavaness, unscathed and so drunk he could hardly stand, kept mumbling that he had insurance, they'd take care of everything. At the hospital he held out for two hours before giving a blood sample. When tested it registered an alcohol level two and a half times the legally permissible amount. Police charged him with drunk driving and a batch of other drink and firearm transgressions. Two weeks later the charge sheet was amended to include a double count of reckless homicide.

In the normal course of events one might expect that causing two deaths by drunk driving would be professional suicide for any physician—but not for Dr. Dale. His patients rallied round the flag and, in a few days, to hear the folks in Eldorado tell it, ole Doc wasn't much more than just the victim of unfortunate circumstances.

Marian couldn't afford to be so charitable. She relinquished forever any idea of reconciliation and decided to move herself and the boys to St. Louis. On the day they were due to leave, Cavaness came grovelling. He pleaded with Marian to stay, to keep the family intact. And then he did something that Marian had never thought him capable of—Dale Cavaness cried.

Marian moved anyway and in December 1971 filed for divorce. The court granted a settlement of $300 a month per child until each was eighteen. Marian received no alimony. She didn't mind. At last she was free. For Cavaness the departure was a minor hiccup. If anything his popularity increased. So did his drinking. He lived at a pace that drew curious glances from interested women and open admiration from most men.

When the reckless driving charges finally came to court in November 1972, Cavaness's team of high-priced lawyers had been indulging in some fancy plea bargaining. Cavaness wound up paying a $1,500 fine and serving three years' probation. In a later civil suit, his insurance company forked over $100,000 to the woman who had survived the accident. She felt abused and bewildered. It didn't seem much for the lives of her husband and baby.

Just over a hundred miles away Marian, too, was undergoing her share of grief. The move to St. Louis hadn't worked out at all the way she had planned or hoped. The boys found difficulty adjusting to their new environment as other children made fun of their rural accents, calling them hicks and rednecks. Mark, in particular, took the move badly and fell in with a tough crowd where drugs were commonplace. His schoolwork deteriorated miserably but paled against the emotional scars he suffered.

Whenever he could the troubled teenager would visit his father in Eldorado, desperate for acceptance. Cavaness hated having him around and used Mark as a punching bag for his drunken spleen. Nothing the boy ever did was good enough. Cavaness belittled him nonstop for his lack of achievement, telling him that he would never amount to anything, never be able to fill his father's shoes. Mark would stand there and take it, tears streaming down his face. A bottomless need to gain his father's acceptance kept him coming back, oblivious to where his tragic persistence was leading him.

Eventually Mark moved back permanently to work for his father as a farmhand. Cavaness paid him two dollars an hour and drove him like a slave. It wasn't much of a life but Mark didn't seem to mind. Cavaness avoided him as much as possible; as far as he was concerned, Mark was hired help, nothing more.

In April 1974 Marian drove down from St. Louis to see Mark for the Easter weekend. Kevin also made the trip from college in Mississippi. Mark was supposed to show up the next day, Good Friday, but didn't. Both Marian and Kevin were surprised; on the phone Mark had sounded really excited about seeing them. When Cavaness arrived next morning there was still no sign of Mark. He claimed not to have seen Mark since the previous Monday. Then, out of the blue, Cavaness dropped a bombshell—he was sure that Mark was dead, a feeling deep inside told him!

Marian and Kevin traded fearful glances. Surely this was just another example of Cavaness's callousness, something designed to hurt and upset them. Wasn't it? They went immediately to the farm.

They found Mark's body lying almost hidden in some grass. At least they thought it was Mark. Wild animals had almost entirely devoured the carcass. Only the distinctive belt buckle and a wallet nearby confirmed their very worst fears. Police summoned to the scene determined that Mark had been shot through the head.

One school of thought sided with the notion that the killing had been accidental. They theorized that Mark had shot himself while reaching inside his truck for a rifle, then his body had been dragged into the long grass by scavenging animals. Other investigators did not credit this. They believed that Mark Cavaness had been murdered.

At around four o'clock Cavaness showed up. He acted like any grieving father, totally distraught, but insistent that it must have been an accident. Later that day Cavaness confided to Marian that, just two months before, he had insured Mark's life for $40,000. She recoiled in horror. Gut instinct told her that Dale Cavaness had killed his own son. Hadn't he always said that, if he caught Mark fooling around with drugs, he'd kill him? But as fast as the idea came Marian discarded it, ashamed of herself for even thinking such a thing; the idea of a father killing his own son was just too foul to consider.

Everyone in Eldorado, except the police, maintained that the death of Mark Cavaness had been an accident. After all, hadn't ole Doc treated them for nothing? Only right to stand behind him.

News of the big insurance policy only reinforced police suspicions about Cavaness. They dug into his background and uncovered a brute always ready to use his fists to settle disputes. His drinking was already notorious following his convictions for reckless homicide but there were other incidents as well: an arrest for brawling in a bar, then wrecking his prison cell. Because he was the town doctor that infraction had been discreetly overlooked. Cavaness, by virtue of his position, was used to getting away with anything; years of uncritical adulation had fostered in him an utter contempt for convention. Detectives knew all this; they also knew that proving Cavaness murdered his son would be one hell of a task.

And so Dr. Dale Cavaness slipped, unblemished, back into the mainstream of town life. His drinking resumed its furious pace. His temper worsened. His sexual appetite became even more voracious. Not even a 1980 conviction for deceptive practices in his job could stop him. Sadly, it only highlighted the shameful bias shown to Cavaness whenever he wound up in trouble. For this felony he was fined $500, ordered to pay $1,700 in restitution and given one year's probation. By contrast, his codefendant was fined a similar amount but hammered with $10,000 in restitution and five years' probation. Cavaness kept his license and kept on practicing, seemingly untouchable.

Other family members weren't so fortunate. Sean, devastated by his brother's death, began drinking heavily. To escape he headed for the Oklahoma oil fields. More disaster awaited him. His arrival coincided with the global downturn in the price of oil. Domestic drilling entered its worst slump in a generation. Rigs shut down, layoffs became commonplace. Newcomers like Sean had two choices: stay and starve, or leave. He chose the latter and slunk, tail between his legs, back to Illinois and the wrath of his father. Cavaness gave him hell for being a failure, driving Sean deeper into the abyss of alcohol abuse.

Finally, in December 1983, he entered a rehabilitation unit in an effort to straighten himself out.

Meanwhile, Cavaness had troubles of his own. He just couldn't control his spending. Without the restraining hand of someone like Eddie Miller, he kept throwing his money into one worthless venture after another. Just when things were at their worst, however, salvation came in the form of another big insurance claim. One of his trailer homes burned to the ground. Had the insurers known that, just prior to the blaze, Cavaness had conveniently removed much of the furniture, they might have been less willing to pay the $100,000 claim.

Cavaness didn't know it, but this insurance swindle came within an inch of undoing him. In an entirely unrelated case, detectives targeting a suspected drug dealer had rigged up a wiretap. The dealer proved to be refreshingly communicative. After mentioning a "Dr. Cavaness" as the source of his morphine, he went on to boast that, just recently, he had done the Doc a favor and set his trailer on fire. Detectives took this information to a local judge and requested a warrant. The judge refused on the grounds that the informant was not a reliable source. Police frustration was tempered by the belief that Cavaness had killed his son, and that one day Dale Cavaness's braggadocio would get the better of him.

All they had to do was wait.

The rehabilitation treatment worked wonders for Sean. Steadily his drinking lessened and he got his life back on track. Oddly enough, his recovery also marked a perceptible change in Dale Cavaness. No longer remote and distant, the father began to exhibit a hitherto unsuspected interest in his sons' welfare. Why, he even took out an investment plan to provide for their future! Ominously, unmentioned and buried deep inside the plan, were yet more insurance policies, payable to himself should any of them die.

By this time Marian had remarried. Sean, determined to show his independence, rented an apartment in St. Louis but had trouble finding a job. As the bills and the pressures mounted, he began sneaking a drink every so often. By December 1984 he was hitting the bottle in a big way. The family talked together on the phone. All of them feared for Sean.

They had no way of knowing just how valid those fears were.

The call came through to Kevin Cavaness on December 13. It was the St. Louis police; Sean had been shot dead. In between sobs, Kevin blurted out that he couldn't believe this nightmare was happening again. Asked to elaborate, he told the police that seven years earlier, he had lost another brother to a bullet. By the end of the call the police were all ears. Like his brother, Sean had also been shot in the head. Similarly, at the time of his death, he was twenty-two, the same age as Mark. Initially the police suspected that they were dealing with some lunatic who had a grudge against the Cavaness family, but interviews with friends who had been with Sean the night before his death revealed an anomaly. According to them he was stone-cold sober, and yet Sean's blood alcohol level showed perilously high levels early next morning when he was found. Where had the booze come from? One possible solution was provided by Sean's neighbors.

They reported seeing a car acting suspiciously outside Sean's apartment at about 10:30 PM. Quite by chance they had taken a note of the license plate. Later they had seen Sean approaching from the direction of a nearby shop. He and the driver of the car had embraced. When the driver stepped into the light from a streetlamp the neighbors recognized him as Dale Cavaness. The two had gone up to Sean's apartment and, judging by the racket, had themselves a fine old time. At some time in the early hours of the morning neighbors heard the two leave.

A check of the license plate confirmed that it did, indeed, belong to Dale Cavaness. Detectives now had definite evidence that Cavaness had been at his son's apartment. It was the kind of break every sleuth dreams about but rarely gets.

Questioned about his whereabouts on the fateful night, Cavaness did something remarkably stupid—he denied ever having been in St. Louis. It was a monumental blunder. After all, what could be more natural than a father visiting his son? Had he said, yes, I saw Sean, but when I left he was just fine, it is difficult to imagine how the police could have proven otherwise. But his denial gave detectives an opening. Acting on Kevin's comments they contacted the Eldorado police and learned of their suspicions regarding the death of Mark Cavaness.

The net drew tighter.

Cavaness, meanwhile, seemed quite unconcerned about the whole affair. His cruel indifference can be gauged by a remark he made to Kevin when the latter waxed nostalgic about his late brother. Cavaness seethed as the eulogy rolled on, until he finally erupted: "Now wait just a moment! Let's not make Sean into something he was not."

"What do you mean by that?" Kevin retorted.

"He was an embarrassment to me."

An icy chill dropped like a guillotine. Kevin stared at his father, unable to believe his own ears. For his part Cavaness just glowered, blue eyes glittering. Even in death, he wasn't about to bestow any compliments on his hated son.

Within days of Sean's funeral, police took Cavaness in for questioning. Confronted by the testimony placing him at Sean's apartment, he continued to deny having been there. One night in the cells changed all that. Okay, he had seen his son that night. He'd denied everything because he didn't want to become a suspect. But, hell, that didn't make him a murderer!

For someone who prided himself on his own cleverness, Cavaness proved remarkably stupid when it came to protecting his interests. Without it being legally necessary, he submitted to a polygraph. Maybe he thought he could beat it. The examiner thought otherwise. According to him, Dale Cavaness was lying through his teeth about what had happened on the night of Sean's death. The police investigation gathered pace. When they discovered the existence of insurance policies totalling $140,000 on Sean's life, that clinched it and Cavaness was charged with first degree murder.

His story continued to change, this time reaching extremes of Gothic fantasy. He and Sean had hit the Mississippi waterfront bars, drinking hard. "What about Sean's alcohol problem?" detectives queried. Cavaness just shrugged. Later they had just cruised around for a while. While driving past some fields, Sean had asked his father to stop the car because he wanted to look at some cows. At the same time, said Cavaness, Sean asked if he could see his .357 Magnum. Cavaness duly handed over the gun, and the two stood for some time watching the cattle. Cavaness had just returned to the car for a can of soda when he heard Sean cry out behind him: "Tell Mom I'm sorry." With the gun at his head, he then squeezed the trigger. Before Cavaness could reach him Sean was dead.

In order to spare Marian the stress and shame of having to deal with suicide, Cavaness said he had picked up the gun and shot Sean in the head again, to make it appear like murder.

Even veteran officers reeled at this. Not one of them could recall such a story being told in such an inhuman manner. In trying to exonerate himself, Cavaness wholly miscalculated the revulsion that he generated—the thought that any father would shoot his own son in the head, just to spare someone's feelings! And to top it all, insulting their intelligence with the absurd notion that two people would stand in the middle of a winter's night just to look at some cows!

When the St. Louis detectives took their suspicions to Southern Illinois, they came up against a brick wall of silence. Folks refused to believe Cavaness capable of killing anyone, let alone his own son. To show their loyalty the local citizenry organized a defense fund for their embattled physician and did everything they could to obstruct the investigation. The fund grew steadily until it amounted to $36,000, all of it raised from friends, patients and employees of Cavaness, each certain he was the victim of some big city frame-up. Frustrated detectives had to content themselves with one thought; at least the killing had taken place in St. Louis—they wouldn't have stood a chance of convicting Cavaness in his home town.

In the face of this reticence the police had to make the case against Cavaness airtight. They found the gun and Sean's belongings where Cavaness said he had left them, on the farm at Harrisburg. Forensic and ballistics experts got together and determined from the position of the wounds and the body that the first shot had to have come from the rear, making suicide virtually impossible. It appeared as though Cavaness had crept up behind Sean, shot him in the back of the head at point-blank range, then once more as he lay on the ground. Nothing else fit the facts.

The trial of Dr. Dale Cavaness began on July 8, 1985 in St. Louis. The prosecution painted a picture of a man plagued by debts of $500,000 and facing financial ruin. Their version of what had happened on that lonely roadside had a father luring his son into the night, then shooting him down for the insurance money. It made for grim listening. But the most compelling testimony against Cavaness came from his own family. Marian and Kevin took the stand and detailed years of abuse, stripping Cavaness bare. All the accused could do was sit and listen and glare. Spectators said that the venom pouring out of Dale Cavaness's icy blue eyes at that moment was something horrible to behold.

With everything proceeding as planned, prosecutors expected to get their hoped-for conviction within a week. But then disaster struck. Somehow Cavaness's polygraph report was inadvertently introduced into evidence. In Missouri, as in most other states, polygraphs are considered too unreliable for court proceedings. These were clear grounds for a mistrial, and the judge so moved.

The prosecution made good use of the hiatus to boost the strength of their forensic case. They enlisted the aid of St. Louis's top forensic pathologist, George Gantner, to examine the evidence and say what he thought. Gantner concluded that the prosecution's case was unassailable.

Because of sensational media coverage, when the second trial convened in November a panel of jurors was brought in from Kansas City to ensure lack of prejudice. Testimony followed much the same course as in the first trial, except that this time Cavaness took the stand. He made a poor witness, cold and far too calculating. Sure, he had money troubles, but no more than the next guy. He glossed over the insurance issue by pointing out that his own life was insured for almost $200,000, with his sons as beneficiaries. Asked why he had shot Sean a second time, Cavaness claimed to have acted on reflexes alone. Odd, said the DA, that he should have remembered to wipe off Sean's hands and then hide the gun while under stress? Cavaness could only bluster. When probed on his son's notorious drinking problem, the defendant protested that he and Sean had actually done very little drinking—manifest nonsense considering the blood-alcohol level in Sean's body. Every sentence that slipped from Cavaness's tongue only damned him further. He shuffled from the stand, discredited and despised.

For months the defense had been casting around for their own ballistics expert, someone to refute the prosecution's case. It proved a thankless task. Most who examined the evidence considered it cast-iron. Finally, an ex-police officer came forward, ready to put his reputation on the line. He offered the court nothing except his belief that the shots had been fired in the order that Cavaness claimed. Under prosecution questioning he conceded that his own experience of bullet wounds on bodies was limited to one short college course. "And who taught that course?" asked the prosecutor. "George Gantner," said the witness. After extracting an eager admission from the ex-cop that Gantner's experience was vastly greater than his own, the prosecution called Gantner to the stand.

The defense moved mountains trying to shake Gantner's testimony but he was rock solid. The shots had to have been fired in the order he said, nothing else matched the evidence. With his own lawyer floundering, Cavaness's bloated ego gave one last manic heave. He demanded the opportunity to cross-examine Gantner himself. The judge and every other court official tried to dissuade Cavaness from such recklessness but their pleas fell on deaf ears. Ignoring the old legal maxim that anyone who defends himself has a fool for a client, Cavaness rose from his seat, confident he could break Gantner.

If there was any lingering doubt in the jury's mind about Cavaness's moral state, then it was destroyed by his demeanor as he locked horns with Gantner. He was just too concerned with demonstrating his own brilliance. Never once did he show any remorse for what had happened. The trial became an excuse for Dale Cavaness to show the world that he was still the tough guy, prepared to fight to the last breath. Except that he had nothing to fight with. Gantner, experienced and massively qualified, tied him up in knots. Cavaness's ploy backfired miserably. The jury could only stare at this extraordinary creature in loathing and amazement. Somehow all the normal emotions had been drained out of Dale Cavaness; they were in the presence of a malignant zombie.

It took the jury just two and a half hours to reach their guilty verdict. A few Cavaness supporters were in court, loyal to the end, cheering loudly as their hero was led away.

Not long afterward Cavaness was back in court for the penalty phase of the trial. After a parade of witnesses had taken the stand to say what a swell guy Dr. Dale was, Kevin stood up and told the world what his father had really been like. The court heard a litany of drunken bullying and brutality almost without parallel. Coming from his own son it was lethal testimony.

American juries generally have been loathe to prescribe the death penalty for members of the medical profession but on this occasion there was no hesitation. They knew they were in the presence of a monster. Acting on their recommendation, the judge sentenced Cavaness to die in the Missouri gas chamber.

Cavaness went off to prison and the customary round of lengthy appeals. He appeared to adjust well to life on death row, getting along with guards and inmates alike. But on the morning of November 17, 1986 a guard conducting the seven o'clock inspection found the lifeless body of Dale Cavaness hanging from his cell door. Around his neck was a noose fashioned from three electrical cords. Right to the very end, Cavaness's will proved indomitable. In order to tighten the noose he had to lean sideways; at any time before losing consciousness he could have reversed the death process by just standing up. Instead, he fought off the survival instinct and died.

It was a remarkable suicide by a remarkable man. A note he left thanked his guards for their kind treatment. Noticeably absent was any reference to his family. When his will was proved the entire proceeds, including the insurance policy, went not to his sons but to a long-time girlfriend.

One last irony: with his final act, Dr. Dale Cavaness still managed to outwit the insurance companies—a clause invalidating his policy should death occur through suicide expired just one day before he hanged himself.

7. A BATTLE OF WILLS

Since its inauguration in 1907 by King Edward VII, London's Central Criminal Court, the Old Bailey, has staged countless criminal trials. Except for the parties concerned, most are of limited interest and rate little more than a paragraph tucked away inside the evening edition, but occasionally a case comes along, so sensational, so unique, that for a few days this magnificent building at the end of Fleet Street becomes the focus of national attention.

Such a trial occurred in April 1957. Beneath the Old Bailey's vaulted ceilings and dazzling frescoes a drama of quite extraordinary dimensions was played out over a period of three weeks. Depending on which version you believed, the defendant was either a man more sinned against than sinning, a victim of horrible circumstances; or he was a mass murderer without precedent. It would be up to the jury to decide.

After just forty-six minutes they were back.

Their faces gave away nothing as they trooped single file to their seats. Reporters in the press box edged forward. The more confident among them already had their story written, although a couple had craftily hedged their bets and scribbled out a quick alternative. You never could tell with juries.

Next came the judge; robed and bewigged, a small sparrow of a man, he was almost lost in the chunky garb of ceremony. His conduct of the long trial had been firm and fair. Whatever the verdict, it was unlikely to suffer condemnation on the grounds of judicial misdirection. He took his seat on the bench.

Almost unnoticed in all this spectacle, as indeed he had been throughout the trial, the defendant readied himself for the verdict. His bulbous, bald head cocked on one side, lips pursed, he stared with owlish intensity through circular wire-rimmed glasses as the clerk of the court rose and spoke.

"Members of the jury, have you reached a verdict?"

The foreman answered, "Yes."

"Do you find the defendant, John Bodkin Adams, guilty or not guilty of murder?"

It was a question that the entire country had been asking for months.

His beginnings were comfortably middle class. His father, a local magistrate in Randallstown, Northern Ireland, also ran a jeweler's shop and John Bodkin Adams was born in the family's first floor flat on January 21, 1899. It was a strict household. His parents belonged to the Plymouth Brethren, rigid fundamentalists who inculcated in their son a respect for the Bible, hard work and money, though not necessarily in that order. Despite the Brethren's doctrine of austerity, Adams was spoiled rotten by his mother who fed him a relentless diet of cream cakes and chocolate. In the process she made her son extremely fat. She also made him devoted to her. It was an attachment that far exceeded normal filial devotion; he became a hopeless "mama's boy." While other children played football in the streets outside, Adams gorged himself on sticky cakes and tagged around the house behind his mother. He was shackled to her and would remain that way for the next forty years.

Toward the end of the First World War he enrolled at Queen's University, Belfast. He wasn't popular with the other students; they found him insufferably pompous and steered well clear of him. An unprepossessing appearance did not help. Less than 5'6" tall, he already tipped the scales at almost two hundred pounds (in later years he would balloon to an even greater bulk), and his face— pink, fleshy and round, and pitted with sharp button eyes—had a repulsive quality that jarred most onlookers.

A fondness for quoting from the scriptures got under people's skin, as did his stuffy disapproval of both alcohol and cigarettes; but what really drove a wedge between Adams and his contemporaries was his morbid preoccupation with money. It dominated his conversation: ways to make it, ways to save it, ways to spend it. At that time, well-bred Britons considered such talk rather bad form; money was fine, of course, but one just didn't harp on about it. Shunned for this reason, Adams fell back on his studies. After qualifying as an MD in 1921, and after one year at a Bristol hospital, he answered a newspaper ad "for a Christian young doctor-assistant" with a large group practice. Adams got the job and packed his bags. His lifelong association with the seaside resort of Eastbourne was about to begin.

Sleepy and slow, Eastbourne has a long tradition of catering for the elderly and the affluent. The mild climate and gentle pace lend themselves easily to bones and minds no longer as flexible as they once were. For a doctor intent on making his mark, Eastbourne might yield a rich harvest. Few could have foreseen the vigor, however, with which Adams would pursue his goals.

He flung himself into his practice. Soon the sight of the fat doctor, chins wobbling over a celluloid collar and perched precariously on his motorcycle, racing to his next appointment, became a common one around Eastbourne. Drive and ambition of this order, rare in such surroundings, made him stand out among fairly languid competition. Patients, especially those with money, began taking him into their confidence. One invited the young physician to attend a shooting party on his estate. Adams jumped at the chance, thus beginning his fascination with shooting and guns.

Adams had no great talent as a physician; indeed, he was infamous for referring even the most mundane cases to other doctors for a second opinion, but his bedside manner was impeccable. Early on he realized that flattery and a sympathetic ear more than compensated for any technical deficiencies. Attention, that was what the wealthy wanted, and he gave it to them in spades, ladling out compliments, worming his way into confidences, wheedling ruthlessly. Elderly ladies loved the way Dr. Adams caressed their hands or brushed their hair. In time most became irrevocably dependent on him, a situation he did nothing to discourage.

As a medical practitioner he was decidedly unorthodox. Frequently, while tending to a patient, he would fall to his knees and pray for divine assistance. The benefits or otherwise of this treatment are unknown but the idiosyncracy endeared him to countless souls, many of whom were, perhaps, not too far distant from meeting their maker and rather cared for this unusual attention to their spiritual well-being. Increasingly they took Adams into their confidence. He had a knack for finding out everything, especially their financial arrangements.

Throughout the thirties he prospered, buying a large rambling house called Kent Lodge and staffing it with a retinue of servants. Always he kept large amounts of money on hand, often running into thousands. A legacy of his childhood, he could never conquer that morbid dread of being poor.

In 1936 he had his one recorded fling with the opposite sex. Norah O'Hara was the daughter of Eastbourne's wealthiest butcher. It seemed like an ideal match. But Adams's mother disapproved of the liaison and on her direction he broke off the engagement. Never again did he venture near the altar. Armchair psychologists have long pondered on Adams's sexuality or lack of it. There was never a breath of scandal attached to his name and the likelihood is that he was simply disinterested.

The outbreak of the Second World War affected him less than most. Age and occupation precluded him from service and left him free to tend his practice. His greatest wartime trauma came, not from any bomb or other enemy action, but rather with the death of his mother in March 1943. At a stroke the great anchor of his life was removed. Despondent and cast adrift, Adams's sole consolation was the knowledge that his mother had bequeathed him £7,043 in her will.

At the end of the war the newly elected Labour Government, with its introduction of the National Health Service, dealt a body blow to Adams and other like-minded medical buccaneers. At a stroke every British citizen was entitled to free medical treatment. Adams responded by whittling down his NHS practice to the minimum allowable and concentrating only on those patients who could afford to pay. It brought handsome rewards: suits from Savile Row, two Rolls Royces, a couple of MGs, a Morris Minor—and several expensive guns.

Rebuked by several colleagues for his rather selective application of the Hippocratic Oath, Adams dismissed their criticism as professional jealousy, remarking to a fellow Irish doctor: "The trouble with you fellows is that you don't know how to make money."

Success followed him into the fifties. He became senior partner in the Dickensian-sounding practice of Adams, Snowball, Harris and Barkworth, and boasted a five-figure income. But tongues were beginning to wag, and not all of it could be dismissed as the envious scuttlebutt of disgruntled fellow physicians.

By late 1956 Eastbourne was awash with rumors about Dr. John Bodkin Adams and the suspiciously high rate of mortality among his patients. Not that gossip about Adams was anything new, the murmurings had begun two decades earlier, in 1935, when one of his patients, Alice Whitton, had died. In Eastbourne, with its elderly population, death was a common occurrence, but what made this particular death noteworthy was that Adams benefitted to the tune of £3,000 under the terms of Mrs. Whitton's will. Citing ethical misconduct, a niece contended the disposition in court, but the judiciary sided with Adams and he was allowed to keep his bequest.

Thus began Adams's long and lucrative career as a legacy hunter. It all stemmed from his singular knack of insinuating himself into the wills of rich patients who rarely lived long afterward. An early conquest was Emily Mortimer. Her family, in an effort to keep its fortune intact, had an unspoken rule that, whenever a relative died, the bulk of the estate was divided among the surviving family members. Under Adams's oily coaxing, Emily broke with tradition. In the year before her death she changed her will twice. First she transferred £3,000 in shares to Adams, then increased the sum to £5,000, all at the expense of her family. When she died, Adams signed her death certificate and pocketed his money.

He did not always meet with unqualified success. When a steel merchant, William Mawhood, who had lent Adams £3,000 to buy a house, lay dying, Adams asked his wife Edith to leave the bedroom for a moment. Puzzled, she lingered by the door and overheard Adams say, "Leave your estate to me and I'll look after your wife." In a fury, Mrs. Mawhood chased the fat physician from the bedroom, hurling her stick after him. Other patients reported similar incidents.

Two elderly ladies were manipulated by Adams into letting him sell their house so that they might move into a smaller, more manageable flat. He then refused to hand over the sale proceeds. Two years and one court order later, they finally got their money.

But it was the wills that intrigued Adams most: Harriet Hughes, sixty-six, was a typical example of the type of person who left him money. Against bank advice she made Adams executor of her estate, then, at his request, added two codicils. The first was that she be cremated. The second, a month later, bequeathed £1,000 each to a Mr. and Mrs. Thurston, friends of Adams. After her death, it was discovered that Adams had actually received 90 percent of the bequests, paying the Thurstons 10 percent for use of their names.

When one patient had the temerity to die without mentioning Adams in her will, he stormed round to her house, squealing, "I deserve something for looking after her!" As astonished mourners looked on, he rummaged through the woman's effects, snatched up a typewriter and some bric-a-brac, threw them into his car and drove off.

Odious and repetitive behavior of this kind could hardly escape attention forever and, inevitably, word of Adams's misconduct reached the local constabulary. It fell to Detective Inspector Brynley Pugh to investigate. What he found disturbed and unnerved him. If only half the stories were true, then not only was Dr. John Bodkin Adams a shameless rogue, but quite possibly the worst murderer in British history. Pugh moved cautiously, sifting through records that went back years. As the whole distasteful story revealed itself, one rumor above all others kept cropping up. It concerned a married couple, both of whom had died while under Adams's care. Pugh decided to look more closely . . .

In 1950 a Mrs. Tomlinson had become Adams's patient after the sudden death of her husband. Still only in her forties, she had taken the bereavement hard and was, according to Adams, depressed and suicidal. Under his treatment she made dramatic progress. Adams introduced her to his own circle of friends, including Jack Hullett, an elderly widower who had also recently lost his spouse. Adams brought Mrs. Tomlinson and Hullett together and, in time, the couple married. Despite the twenty-year disparity in their ages, they lived happily together. Both continued to receive treatment from Adams. He described them as being very nervous, and much of the medication he prescribed was in the form of sedatives.

In November 1955 Hullett went into hospital for a serious operation. At Christmas he was well enough to return home and was nursed there under Adams's supervision. On March 13, 1956, Hullett and his wife, together with the nurse, went out to a local pub for a drink.

All three came home for dinner. Later Hullett complained of feeling "breathless." As this often occurred after bouts of exertion the nurse wasn't unduly concerned but still thought it best to telephone Adams. He arrived at 8:30 PM. First he examined Hullett, who said that he was suffering from a "bad headache," then helped him upstairs to his bedroom. When the night nurse came on duty she found Hullett "flopped in his chair," but heard him tell Adams that he felt all right. Adams briefed the nurse, then left to get medication. He returned at 10:30 PM. Hullett, by now in bed, was still awake. Adams administered an injection of morphine and Hullett fell asleep. With his patient resting peacefully, Adams left.

At 6 AM Hullett awoke, asked the time, told his nurse that there was nothing he wanted and fell asleep again. Half an hour later he died. Adams was summoned and gave the cause of death as cerebral hemorrhage accompanied by coronary thrombosis.

Jack Hullett died a wealthy man, leaving £94,644. Apart from a few small bequests, including £500 to Adams, the residue went to his widow. In accordance with his fondness for hastening funeral formalities, Adams neglected to mention the £500 when signing the cremation form. Not only was this unethical but it was also illegal. Under British law no physician can sign a cremation order if he or she has any financial interest in the death of the deceased. Over the years this was a convention that Adams flouted repeatedly.

Adams continued to attend Mrs. Hullett. Widowed for the second time in just a few years, her depression deepened. Adams recommended that she consult a psychiatrist. When she refused, he increased her medication to two tablets of sodium barbiturate a day.

In July of 1956 Mrs. Hullett engaged in a flurry of activity. On the twelfth she had a new will drawn up by her solicitors. Under its terms her entire estate, net value £137,302, went to her family, apart from half a dozen specific bequests, one of which was a Rolls Royce for Adams.

She also dealt with one other piece of unfinished business. Apparently her husband had promised Adams a car but had neglected to make such provision in his will. In lieu of the car Mrs. Hullett offered Adams a cash settlement. He accepted. On Tuesday, July 17, she drew a check in Adams's favor for £1,000. The next day Adams deposited the check at his bank and inquired when it would be cleared. The cashier told him the twenty-first. Adams asked if it could be cleared sooner. Only if specially presented, said the cashier. Adams requested that this be done and the check was cleared on July 19.

That very evening Mrs. Hullett went to bed early, complaining of a headache. At about 10 PM she swallowed a massive overdose of barbiturates, 115 gm, and fell into a coma.

Next morning, at 8 AM, the maid took in Mrs. Hullett's orange juice. Her mistress didn't stir. An hour later the maid returned with the breakfast tray. Still Mrs. Hullett hadn't moved. When Adams called at his usual time, he opened the bedroom door a fraction, listened to her breathing, declared it normal and did not disturb her. At 12:15 PM the maid entered the bedroom and drew the curtains but Mrs. Hullett slept on. By 3 PM the maid was worried enough to ring Adams's surgery. Adams, who was at a meeting, received the message and told the receptionist to send his partner, Dr. Harris, saying that he would go just as soon as he got back.

Harris arrived at 3:30 PM to find Mrs. Hullett comatose. Hearing that she had complained of headache and some giddiness, he diagnosed possible cerebral hemorrhage. But one thing troubled him. According to the maid, Adams had been giving Mrs. Hullett sleeping pills every night, yet Harris could not find an empty bottle. After giving Mrs. Hullett an injection, he left.

Adams arrived an hour later and telephoned for Harris to return. The two discussed Mrs. Hullett's condition. Harris mentioned a possible drug overdose. Adams shook his round, bald head: no, not possible. He also pooh-poohed Harris's suggestion that they obtain another opinion. Next day, though, Adams rang a consultant named Dr. Shera and asked him to perform various tests. Shera asked if the patient was on barbiturates. Adams replied affirmatively and signed a request for an analysis of the urine to be tested for an excess of barbiturates.

On the Saturday afternoon Adams went to the local hospital to get some megimide, an antidote for barbiturate poisoning. The manufacturers' instructions called for 3–5 ccs to be given every five minutes until recovery. Usually this meant a total dosage of between 100 and 200 ccs, but Adams neglected to read the instructions. Instead, he asked a house surgeon what the normal dose was. The doctor told him to give 10 ccs only. If that didn't work, further doses would be futile.

For two days Adams stayed with his patient, getting up in the middle of the night to give Mrs. Hullett a multitude of injections. Despite this she died early on Monday morning, July 23. At this point, Adams's earlier urgency at the bank assumes a new and possibly sinister significance.

Ordinarily the check he presented would have been cleared on July 21. Had Adams known or suspected on the eighteenth that Mrs. Hullett was about to attempt suicide, and had he provided the means by which she might accomplish this, then he must also have recognized the likelihood that she would be dead by the twenty-first (in which case the check would not clear at all). Requesting an accelerated clearance ensured that the funds were safely in his own account, come what may. This incident was just one in a series of inconsistencies which hinted that all was not straightforward in the death of Mrs. Hullett. There had already been others.

While Mrs. Hullett was comatose, Harris told Adams that if she died a postmortem would be necessary. Adams blanched and wondered if this could be done privately. Early on Sunday morning he rang the coroner to make inquiries. The coroner, astonished to hear that the patient had not yet died, brusquely advised Adams that such a request was both insensitive and premature. After death, he said, the ordinary notification should be given. Then he hung up. Adams, possibly realizing the precarious nature of his position, next drafted an odd letter for himself and Harris to sign. Not so much a formal report, it was more an account of who said what to whom; it reeked of someone anxious to cover his tracks. In it he emphasized how strictly he had prescribed barbiturates to Mrs. Hullett: "She could not possibly have secreted any of this."

That day the coroner, after consulting the chief constable, formally opened an inquest. It was adjourned to await the results of a postmortem. A statement to this effect, communicated to local newspapers, was snatched up by Fleet Street. Next day, a tidal wave of reporters engulfed Eastbourne and, when the inquest resumed on August 21, there was hardly a person in the country who did not know of Dr. John Bodkin Adams.

The coroner raised a number of questionable points. Knowing of Mrs. Hullett's suicidal tendencies, he asked Adams, what precautions did you take? Adams replied that he personally dispensed just two tablets a day, a total of 15 gm. The coroner pressed. Did Adams know that 50 gm of sodium barbiturates taken all at once could be a fatal dose? Adams said that he did. Then how, asked the coroner, had Mrs. Hullett been able to acquire the 115 gm, or eight days' supply, that killed her?

Whenever he was asked a particularly difficult question, Adams had a habit of rolling his eyes back so that only the whites were visible. This was such an occasion. Quickly he stammered that Jack Hullett had also taken barbiturates and that after his death no steps had been taken to retrieve any surplus. Perhaps Mrs. Hullett had hoarded these tablets?

Another possibility emerged when Adams admitted that, before going on holiday in June, he had given Mrs. Hullett thirty-six tablets to cover his absence. Yet, asked about his reaction to the news on July 20 that Mrs. Hullett was seriously ill, Adams claimed that the prospect of barbiturate poisoning never entered his mind: "I thought I had the tablets tightly cleared up."

By any reckoning, Adams's performance was weak. He gave the impression of a doctor either criminally negligent or else criminally inclined. To the surprise of onlookers, however, the jury returned a verdict of suicide. This didn't prevent reporters from indulging in an orgy of speculation. Headlines screamed that Scotland Yard detectives were investigating the possible mass poisoning of wealthy victims in Eastbourne during the past twenty years—as many as four hundred!

Such hostile publicity and the mere mention of Scotland Yard would have unnerved most men, but not Dr. Adams. One day after the inquest Percy Hoskins, chief crime reporter of the *Daily Express*, and Adams's only Fleet Street ally, travelled up to London with the doctor on the train from Eastbourne. He found him quite unconcerned, and his warning to Adams that he was in serious danger made little impression.

The two Scotland Yard detectives delegated to investigate Adams were Superintendent Herbert Hannam and Sergeant Charles Hewitt. Though facing an enormous task, Hannam was not a man plagued by self-doubt. On the contrary, his reputation was one of vast self-assurance. A penchant for expensive suits and big cigars had earned him the nickname of "The Count." Unlike many policemen, he felt comfortable with the press and they courted him assiduously. Hannam felt certain that he could nail Dr. John Bodkin Adams; all it would take was some good, old-fashioned detective work.

An army of assistants began searching the official records at Somerset House. It was dry, laborious work but fruitful as they uncovered the astounding fact that Adams had been a legatee in no less than 132 wills! Furthermore, a disproportionally high number of the deceased had been cremated. In total it made for damning suspicion but was not, under British law, terribly useful. Crown policy at that time eschewed multiple murder indictments. The feeling was that anyone accused of murder should only have to defend himself against one charge at a time. Hannam's duty was to find that one charge.

Remorselessly Hannam pruned away at the rumors and hearsay until he was left with a dozen possibilities. On October 1, 1956, he and the doctor had their first meeting, just as Adams was putting his car in the garage. It began in best detective-story style with Hannam stepping out of the evening gloom and inquiring politely: "Good evening, doctor. Did you have a good holiday in Scotland?"

Adams eyed the tall, elegant police officer for a moment. He must have expected this, but any nerves were well concealed. The two men introduced themselves and the duel began. Adams, a compulsive talker, blabbed freely. After detailing his Scottish shooting trip, he went on, without prompting, to give a general account of his life, one that heavily emphasized his religious commitment, declaring that it was God's guidance that had brought him to Eastbourne.

Hannam mentioned the rumors which were flying all over town. Adams rolled his eyes, sighing, "I think it is all God's plan to teach me a new lesson," he said. "I gave a vow to God that I would look after my national poor patients, day and night I will turn out for them . . . I think this makes people jealous of me."

But what about all those legacies?

"A lot of those were instead of fees. I don't want money," he scoffed. "What use is it? I paid £1,100 supertax last year."

Grilled about a chest of silver that Mrs. Hullett had owned, Adams said, "Mrs. Hullett was a very dear patient. She insisted a long time before she died that I should have that in her memory . . . I knew she was going to leave it to me, and her Rolls Royce."

Conversation turned to Jack Hullett and the bequest of £500. "There is no mystery about him," said Adams. "He told me long before his death that he had left me money in his will. I even thought that it would have been more than it was . . . I have one thing in life and God knows I have vowed to Him I would—that is, to relieve pain and let these dear people live as long as possible." Attempting to gloss over his improper cremation procedure, Adams cooed, "Oh, that wasn't done wickedly . . . We always want cremations to go off smoothly for the dear relatives. If I said I knew I was getting money under the will, they might get suspicious and I like cremations and burials to go smoothly. There was nothing suspicious really. It wasn't deceitful."

Hannam drove off into the night, exasperated and nauseated by Adams's sanctimonious moralizing. He was also convinced that he had just spoken to a murderer.

On November 24, armed with a search warrant issued under the Dangerous Drugs Act, Hannam returned. By this time the case had achieved international celebrity. British newspapermen now had to compete with their counterparts from the USA and Europe for scraps of news. Camped outside Kent Lodge, they made such a commotion that Hannam ordered all the blinds to be closed; this only heightened journalistic speculation. Right from the outset Hannam had kept the press unusually well informed in the hope that their incessant presence would get the doctor to crack.

Adams proved equal to the task. He told Hannam, "There is no question of a statement, for I have been told not to make one."

Then he proceeded to talk his head off.

Asked about morphine and heroin he said, "You will find none here . . . I very, very seldom use them." Hannam asked to see his drug register, the record doctors are supposed to keep, showing the disbursement of any dangerous drugs, Adams feigned ignorance. "I don't know what you mean. I keep no register."

Hannam pressed about some prescriptions written for another patient, a Mrs. Edith Morrell, who had died some years earlier. "Were there any [tablets] left over when she died?"

"No, none. All were given to the patient."

"Doctor, you prescribed for her seventy-five heroin tablets days before she died."

"Poor soul, she was in terrible agony. It was all used, I used them myself . . . Do you think it was too much?'

Hannam icily replied that that was not for him to say and ordered his men to begin searching the surgery. Adams remained in the room while they did so. As the search advanced to some cupboards on either side of the fireplace he became increasingly agitated. While one was being searched he sidled over to the other and with a key unlocked a compartment and removed two items. Hannam saw him.

"What did you take from that cupboard, doctor?"

"Nothing, I only opened it for you."

"You put something into your pocket."

"No, I've got nothing."

"What was it, doctor?"

Sheepishly, Adams produced two bottles of hyperduric morphine. Hannam said, "Doctor, please don't do silly things like that. It is against your own interests."

"I know it was silly. I didn't want you to find it in there."

Two days later Adams was arrested and brought before magistrates on thirteen minor offenses related to the misuse of dangerous drugs and contravening the Cremation Act of 1902. The charges were cosmetic. The main object of the exercise was to confiscate Adams's passport; the police didn't want him making a run for it.

The task of building a substantial murder charge against Adams was orchestrated by Hannam and Hewitt in conjunction with the attorney general, Reginald Manningham-Buller, and the director of public prosecutions, Sir Edwin Matthews. The case that Hannam thought the strongest involved Clara Neil-Miller. A fellow patient in the nursing home, where Miss Neil-Miller resided, had told how

> Dr. Adams was called in one night in February 1954. She [Miss Neil-Miller] had either a severe cold or flu. He remained in her bedroom for nearly forty-five minutes before leaving. I later became worried as I heard nothing from the room. I opened the door and was horrified at what I saw. This was a bitterly cold winter's night. The bedclothes on her bed had been pulled back and thrown over the bed-rail at the base. Her nightdress had been folded back across her body up to her neck. All the bedroom windows had been flung open. A cold gush of wind was sweeping through the bedroom. That is how the doctor left her.

The next day Clara Neil-Miller died, leaving Adams £5,000 in her will. In addition she had recently paid him two checks for £500 and £300 for reasons unknown. After interviewing the nursing home proprietress, Mrs. Elizabeth Sharp (who knew Adams's practice inside out), Hannam was confident that she would tell all. But Matthews and Manningham-Buller dithered and, when the detectives returned to Eastbourne, Mrs. Sharp was dead and cremated. Very convenient, thought Hannam. Very convenient.

Frustrated but not beaten, Hannam and Hewitt met Manningham-Buller at the House of Commons. To their dismay he ordered them to proceed on the Edith Morrell case. Both argued that a much stronger case could be made against Adams on the two Hullett deaths. But the attorney general was not a man easily deflected from a decision once made. Not for nothing had he earned the nickname Reginald "Bullying-Manner." Morell it would be. Hannam and Hewitt left the meeting gloomy and pessimistic.

On December 19 they traveled to Eastbourne and arrested Adams for the murder of Edith Alice Morrell. His reaction was astonishment: "Murder? Can you prove it was murder?"

Hannam replied, "You are now charged with murdering her."

"I did not think that you could prove murder," Adams said. "She was dying in any event."

When the receptionist brought Adams his coat he clutched her hand and said, "I will see you in Heaven."

Until that happy day dawned John Bodkin Adams had to be content with Brixton Prison in South London. There he spent 111 days on remand as Inmate 7889 until his trial at the Old Bailey.

At the committal proceedings, Adams was indicted on three counts of murder, the Hulletts and Edith Morell, though the Crown intended to proceed only on the latter charge. Hannam had good reason to feel despondent about the Morrell case, it had all happened so long ago . . .

In June 1948 Edith Morrell, seventy-nine, the wealthy widow of a Liverpool businessman, had suffered a paralyzing stroke. She began her convalescence at an Eastbourne nursing home under the care of Dr. Adams. Mrs. Morrell's irascibility did not endear her to the other patients and few were displeased when she left and took a house of her own. With her considerable fortune she was able to afford an army of nurses to tend to her every whim. Cantankerous and vituperative, Edith Morrell was one of those malcontents whose sole enjoyment comes from making everyone else's life a misery. Her employees loathed her, but she paid well. More resilient than most was the ever-pleasant Dr. Adams. All through 1950 he called regularly. His treatment was simple and effective—ply Mrs. Morrell with enough heroin and morphine to keep her stupefied. In the ten months preceding her death in November 1950, Adams wrote prescriptions for heroin that exceeded the recommended maximum daily dose by 70 percent.

Had Mrs. Morrell been in pain, this blatant overdosing would have been understandable, but the fact remains that she was in no discomfort at all. Authorities believed that Adams was systematically striving to gain control of Mrs. Morrell's will power for his own ends.

On April 28, 1949, Adams had telephoned her solicitor, a Mr. Sogno, saying that she was anxious to change the contents of her will immediately. That day Mr. Sogno went to see his client and she did make another will. In it she bequeathed to Adams a small oak chest containing a silver tea service.

Almost a year passed. In March 1950 Dr. Adams showed up, unannounced, at Mr. Sogno's office. He told Sogno that Mrs. Morrell had promised him her Rolls Royce and also some jewelry but had forgotten to make such provision in her will. Although Mrs. Morrell was seriously ill, Adams said, her mental faculties were in no way impaired and she was well enough to execute a codicil. Sogno hedged. Because of the jewelry's value he suggested waiting until the following weekend (when Mrs. Morrell's son was at home) before making such an amendment. Adams flew into a rage, insisting that the codicil be executed right away, barking that if it didn't meet with the son's approval the codicil could be torn up later.

Edith Morrell seems to have been an inveterate will maker. On July 19, 1950, she added a codicil that, if her son predeceased her, everything would pass to Adams. Just over two weeks later, she again amended her will; this time Adams would receive only the silver chest, the Rolls Royce and an Elizabethan cupboard. In September she was at it again. Furious because Adams had gone away on holiday and left her in the care of his partner, Dr. Harris, Mrs. Morrell executed yet another codicil. In this she revoked all previous gifts to Adams. When the doctor returned from holiday, he learned of the changes and speedily set about restoring himself in Mrs. Morrell's good graces. He succeeded. On October 23 her son, Claude, returned the codicil to Sogno in pieces. Clearly everyone thought that Adams was once again included in the will. He certainly thought so himself, unaware that under British law the mere act of destruction does not nullify a codicil.

On November 13, 1950, Edith Morell died after receiving massive doses of opiates. Although not legally bound to do so, Claude Morrell gave Adams the Rolls Royce. Adams always believed that the car had come to him under the terms of Mrs. Morrell's will. Now it would be up to the Crown to demonstrate that John Bodkin Adams had precipitated the execution of that will.

It has long been the custom in England for the attorney general personally to prosecute any murder case involving the use of poison. In taking on this responsibility Manningham-Buller was not merely following precedent. A career lawyer and politician, he knew that securing a conviction against Adams would greatly enhance his prospects of assuming the mantle of lord chief justice, due to become available soon. Large, bluff and dogmatic to the point of obstinacy, Manningham-Buller chose to ignore obvious deficiencies in the Morrell case—not least the fact that she had died and been cremated six years ago—in favor of a belief that, once on the stand, Adams would convict himself out of his own mouth.

By contrast the counsel briefed to defend Adams was relatively unknown. Geoffrey Lawrence had made his reputation in civil law where he was respected as a dangerously skilled cross-examiner, not someone who badgered witnesses but rather coaxed answers from them. If Manningham-Buller carried the bludgeon, then Lawrence wielded a razor-sharp rapier. It promised to be a memorable contest.

Further stimulus was provided by a recent change in the law. The Homicide Act of 1957, which categorized murder into capital and non-capital offences, had surprisingly excluded poisoning from the list of death-penalty crimes. Passing into law on March 21, three days after the commencement of Adams's trial, the Act was not retroactive; this meant that, if convicted, Adams would be sentenced to death, although the sentence would almost certainly be commuted. But there was one other important consideration. The new act also mandated death for anyone found guilty of murder on two separate occasions. Therefore, should Adams be convicted of killing Mrs. Morell he might then be charged with murdering the Hulletts. At that time Manningham-Buller, a staunch advocate of capital punishment, would doubtless spare no effort in attempting to put a rope around Adams's plump neck.

Manningham-Buller's ferocious determination to secure a conviction became beacon clear when he baldly announced that no evidence pertaining to the Hullett cases would be heard during Adams's trial for killing Mrs. Morrell. Lawrence was furious. He knew just how feeble the Hullett indictments were. Now he had to contend with a jury which knew of other charges pending against the accused but which would never hear just how flimsy those charges were. To say the least it was a low blow.

When the trial began, Manningham-Buller, in legal parlance, "opened high." In broad strokes he painted a lurid picture of a fiend who admitted dispensing massive amounts of dangerous drugs to an elderly patient and who stood to benefit financially from that patient's death. He told the court that he would produce nurses and doctors whose testimony could lead to only one conclusion—that Dr. Adams intended to kill Edith Morrell and profit from her death.

First came the nurses, four of them. Nurse Stronach was the first, telling how, six years earlier, she had seen Dr. Adams give drugs to Mrs. Hullett even though she was comatose. Stronach was adamant: the doctor had repeatedly administered drugs to a woman who was "semiconscious and rambling."

Lawrence began cross-examination gently, bemoaning the passage of time, but Stronach robustly maintained that her memory on the matter was crystal clear. She did, however, admit that a contemporary record had been kept of all treatment, doctors' visits and medicines prescribed. Unfortunately such records were only kept for two years.

"If only," Lawrence sighed, "we had got those reports now, we could see the truth of exactly what happened night by night and day by day."

Stronach, who didn't take kindly to having her recollection questioned, became defiant. "Yes," she snapped. "But you have our word for it."

Whereupon Lawrence reached for an item on his desk, then handed it to the witness. "I want you to look at that book, please."

Every drop of color drained from Stronach's face. Hand trembling, she took the book, the very record that Lawrence had been talking about. A gasp filled the court. Lawrence's team had found what Scotland Yard had not, tucked away in the back of a filing cabinet at Adams's surgery. For the first of several times it looked very much as though the prosecution's case had been hasty and incomplete.

The contemporary record was virtually a direct contradiction of everything that Stronach had said. Far from being "semiconscious and rambling," Mrs. Hullett was described as "bright and not confused and eating a hearty lunch."

"Isn't that what you wrote at the time?"

"I have nothing to say," Stronach mumbled.

"What?"

"I have nothing to say."

"You have nothing to say?"

"No."

Stronach limped from the witness box, shorn of all credibility, to be replaced by Sister Mason-Ellis. She too, was led a merry dance by Lawrence until the overnight adjournment came to her aid.

Normally the recess is a boon to flustered witnesses; they have time to gather their thoughts and perhaps better prepare themselves for the onslaught to come—but not on this occasion. When Sister Mason-Ellis resumed her evidence the next morning Lawrence demanded to know whether she and two other nurses, including Stronach, had been discussing the case together overnight? How Lawrence came by this information remained a mystery for years, but it appears that a fellow passenger, traveling back to Eastbourne on the same train as the three nurses the night before, had overheard them discussing the case.

Next morning he saw them again, this time on the platform at Eastbourne, awaiting the London train, and he distinctly heard one of the nurses remark, "Don't you say that or you'll get me into trouble." Outraged by such connivance, the eavesdropper had contacted Lawrence.

Shamefacedly, the Sister agreed that it was true. Asked what she had been told not to say that very morning, she retorted primly, "Really, I cannot remember because I was not terribly interested, if I may say so."

Lawrence pounced: "I am not asking you to remember something which happened six years ago, as the Attorney General did yesterday!"

It was the coup de grâce. The sister withered under Lawrence's bombardment. Only a fraction of the drugs prescribed were actually given and nothing the nurses said squared with their written record. So emphatic was Lawrence's victory on this point that many expected the Crown to withdraw its case but Manningham-Buller plowed on, convinced that, as soon as he got Adams in the witness box, the doctor's notoriously loose tongue would hang him. Also, the Crown had lined up two of the country's most eminent physicians with expertise in the area of opiates. Surely the jury would heed them.

Dr. Arthur Douthwaite had offices in Harley Street and exuded an aura of science and certitude. The prescriptions written by Adams for Mrs. Morrell, he said, were capable of only one interpretation—on November 8, 1950, Adams formed the intention to "terminate her life" and carried that intention into effect over the next five days. Some of Douthwaite's lofty confidence began to fray as Lawrence drew the grudging admission that, yes, another doctor might study the same data and reach an entirely different conclusion. The longer Douthwaite remained on the stand, the more he shifted his ground. When Lawrence ruthlessly exposed these inconsistencies, Douthwaite, by now visibly shaken, conceded that his earlier evidence was mistaken. Now he thought that Adams had been trying to commit murder from November 1! He compounded this astonishing volte-face by proclaiming that anyone who disagreed with him could not honestly hold such an opinion and was, by implication, a liar. It was a hopelessly inept performance. Expert witnesses are supposed to be firm and resolute. Douthwaite was neither. He came off as pompous, opinionated and wholly feckless.

He was followed by Dr. Michael Ashby. After the mauling dished out to his colleague, Ashby did not seem to have an opinion on anything. Circumspect when he should have been sure, he refused to commit himself one way or the other.

At the conclusion of his case, Manningham-Buller must have surveyed the wreckage around him and cringed. He had seen an already marginal case reduced to rubble. With his career in jeopardy, all hopes were now pinned on crucifying Adams in cross-examination. Because the accused is always the first person called by the defense, everyone in court braced themselves for the imminent confrontation.

Lawrence rose to his feet. "I call Dr. Harman."

There was pandemonium. Reporters rushed for the exits. Unbelievably, John Bodkin Adams was not giving evidence on his own behalf! With one stroke Lawrence had pulled the rug from beneath the prosecutor's feet.

Manningham-Buller sat dumbstruck. For months he had awaited this moment, the chance to expose Adams to the world as a grasping, callous murderer, and now that opportunity was to be denied to him. The prosecution's handling of its case had been so feeble that Adams had no need to argue for his life.

Lawrence was no fool. He knew that the only way he could lose this case was if Adams said something foolish from the witness box. Far better to run the risk of the jury looking unfavorably on any man who would not face his accusers than have Adams destroy everything with a couple of injudicious phrases.

The evidence that Dr. Harman gave directly contradicted that of the Crown doctors and the case soon went to the judge's summing-up. Speaking to the jury, Justice Devlin stressed that they were to ignore the fact that Adams had chosen not to give testimony. It was his right under law and one that should be stoutly maintained. The onus was on the prosecution to prove their case beyond a reasonable doubt and Devlin left little doubt that he felt the Crown had come up several yards short. The jury agreed. After less than a hour's deliberation they returned a verdict of not guilty.

So complete had been the rout that Manningham-Buller said that the Crown would not be proceeding with the other murder charges. John Bodkin Adams was free to go.

He promptly sold his story to the *Daily Express*, the one newspaper that had stuck by him. They paid £10,000 for the privilege. From all accounts this sum covered the costs of Adams's legal expenses. But he wasn't out of the woods yet. He still had to face those charges of contravening the Dangerous Drugs Act. Adams entered a guilty plea and was fined £2,400. In November 1957 he was struck off the Medical Register.

Four years later his license to practice was reinstated, although his authority to prescribe dangerous drugs remained in limbo. Many of his patients remained faithful to him; some still included him in their wills. That same year

Adams won several libel suits against those newspapers that had defamed him and received several thousands of tax-free pounds. Thereafter Adams kept a vigilant eye on the press. As late as 1969, when his name cropped up jokingly in an unrelated article, he sued and was awarded another £500.

Adams remained in Eastbourne and was a founding member of the southeast branch of the Clay Pigeon Shooting Association. Ultimately he became senior honorary life vice-president. His shooting prowess took him to competitions in Oslo, Monte Carlo and Lisbon. He spent much of his later years avoiding the press and lived quietly without a hint of impropriety against his name. Following a fall, he contracted pneumonia and died on July 4, 1983, at the age of eighty-four. All those years of scrimping and saving had been good to him. The most notorious legacy hunter of all left no less than £402,970 in his own will. He bequeathed it to those who had stood by him during his trial.

So was Adams a deliberate murderer who killed for money? Or was he, in his own words, just "easing the passing"? No one will ever know for sure. Most who met him, including his own defense counsel, were sickened by his humbug and greed, and had little difficulty believing him capable of murder. But few could deny that, under the legal niceties of the time, he was rightfully acquitted.

Nowadays he might not have fared so well. The Crown's antipathy to multiple murder charges has diminished and there are only so many coincidences that a jury will stomach. Scotland Yard remained convinced that Adams poisoned at least a dozen, probably more, patients in order to gain a pecuniary advantage. Had the jury heard all the accumulated evidence, then perhaps their decision might have been different, more in line with that of a woman who, just before the trial, was having her hair cut in a fashionable London salon. Turning to the other customers she remarked, "Adams is as guilty as hell—but my husband will get him off." Thus spake Mrs. Lawrence, wife of Adams's defending counsel, Geoffrey Lawrence. Prophetic words, and probably true words as well.

8. KILLING TIME

Among crime aficionados the Wallace Case*—with its baffling telephone call, brutal wife-murder, a husband's suspicious-sounding alibi and trenchant police efforts to undermine the chronology of that alibi—has become a classic of British criminology, the standard by which all other murder mysteries are judged. Many call it unique. Few know, however, that 4,000 miles and almost four decades away from Liverpool, a remarkably similar set of circumstances conspired together on a frigid Illinois morning at the home of a Chicago doctor; the outcome of this provoked a controversy every bit as divisive, every bit as enduring as the Wallace classic. In essence the crimes were identical. So were the doubts surrounding the husband's story.

But there was something else as well, something that a

---

*In 1931 William Wallace, a Liverpool insurance agent, was found guilty of murdering his wife and sentenced to hang. He was later freed when the Appeal Court quashed his conviction on the grounds that it was not supported by the weight of evidence.

nondescript Liverpool insurance agent could never have envisaged; an incredible dash for freedom, brushes with African dictators, illegal passports, Marxist revolutionaries, midnight escapes to safety, and any amount of media hype. At times, the saga reads like a best-selling thriller. But this story is true—every word of it.

The morning of December 22, 1967, broke clear and icy cold in Chicago. The weatherman promised a dry day but not much more; an eviscerating wind off Lake Michigan would see to that. At 9 AM Dr. John Marshall Branion, Jr. left his home in Hyde Park and drove south on Woodlawn Avenue. With him in the car was his four-year-old son, John III. Middle-class, black, undeniably successful, Dr. Branion steered his car along quiet streets untroubled by the race riots that had gutted the South and West Sides of Chicago just months earlier. Hyde Park was an upwardly mobile, cosmopolitan community that cared less about color and more about achievement. Many of its residents either studied or worked at the nearby University of Chicago. As Branion skirted the brick-built campus—birthplace of nuclear-chain reaction—he was aware of how the university threw its shadow across the entire community. He also knew the benefits that accrued to the bright and the ambitious . . . people like himself. At the age of forty-one, Dr. John Marshall Branion, Jr. was plump and he was prosperous, someone on the fast track, blessed with a loving wife and fine children, a model of African-American accomplishment.

Or so it seemed.

After a few minutes' drive he braked to a halt outside the Hyde Park Neighborhood Club, a nursery school approximately one mile from his home. Each weekday morning before work, Branion would drop his son off at the school. Today was no different. He waved good-bye to John, then drove back the way he had come. He retraced his route exactly, passing his house on his way to Ida Mae Scott Hospital. Although by speciality a gynecologist, Branion practiced general medicine at the hospital and this morning he was scheduled to make his normal rounds. Coworkers thought highly of Branion, patients loved him, though some noticed this morning that the doctor did seem a little less jovial than normal, more distracted, as though he had something on his mind.

While Dr. Branion made his rounds, back home his wife, Donna, was putting the final touches to her Christmas preparations. A handsome woman, just now moving into middle age, she and the children had already hung the decorations. Now she was busy alone in the front living room, piling presents around the foot of the tree. Despite the central heating, she wore good warm clothes, her favorite beige sweater and a brown-and-white plaid skirt. Around 10:15 AM she took a break to telephone her sister, Joan Tyler, the second time she'd called that day. The two chatted for several minutes about this and that, the forthcoming holidays and babysitting; then Donna hung up. On the phone she sounded perfectly normal, without a care in the world, so her sister would say later. After the call Donna went back to her festive preparations. Beyond the window, Hyde Park was also gearing up for Christmas . . . a happy time of year.

The Branions fit easily into the community. Donna came from one of Chicago's most prominent black families. Her father and uncles were respected lawyers and businessmen, while first cousin Oscar Brown, Jr., a well-known singer, had an eclectic blend of jazz and folk which brought him into close contact with Bob Dylan. She had

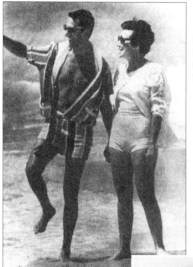

Carl Coppolino relaxing on a Florida beach with his wife during the second trial.

Charles Friedgood—
a career of malpractice that culminated in murder.
Photograph courtesy of the Nassau County Police Department

Except where noted, all photos are in the public domain.

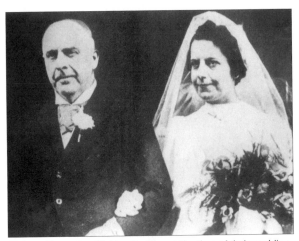

Robert Clements with his wife, Vee, at the time of their wedding.
She would be his fourth victim.

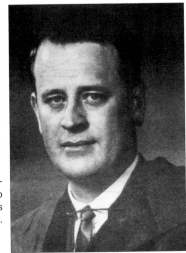

John Hill—
the music-loving gigolo
with a fondness
for deadly pastries.

Except where noted, all photos are in the public domain.

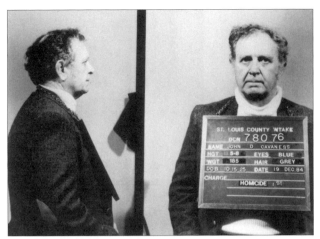

Dale Cavaness murdered two sons for insurance payouts.
Photograph courtesy of the St. Louis Police Department

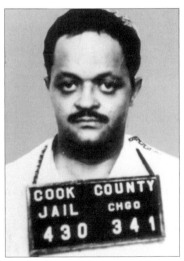

John Branion—
fugitive on the run.
Photograph courtesy of the FBI

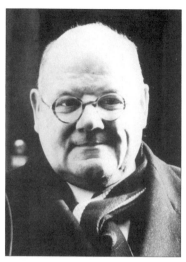

John Bodkin Adams was mentioned in 132 wills.

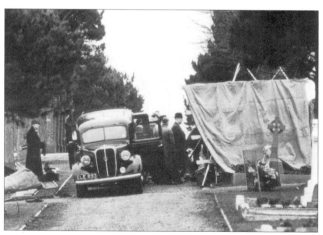

John Bodkin Adams—the exhumation of one suspected victim.

Except where noted, all photos are in the public domain.

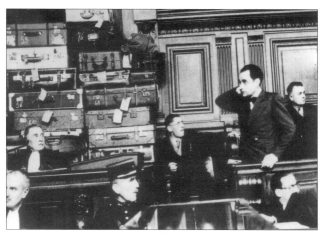

Marcel Petiot—he had no answer for the damning pile of luggage.

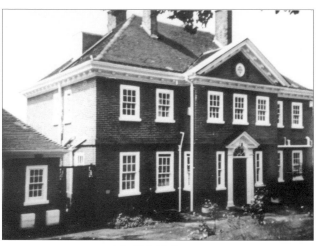

John Baksh's house,
bought with the profits from his first wife's murder.
Photo courtesy of author's collection

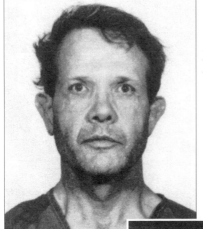

Richard Boggs—
sex, drugs, and money
troubles drove him
to murder.
*Photograph courtesy of the
Glendale Police Department*

John Barrett Hawkins—
the hustler supreme.
*Photograph courtesy of the
Glendale Police Department*

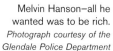

Melvin Hanson—all he
wanted was to be rich.
*Photograph courtesy of the
Glendale Police Department*

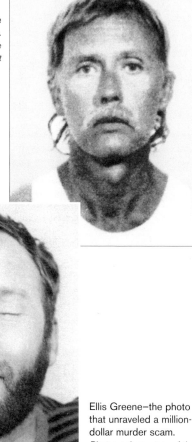

Ellis Greene—the photo
that unraveled a million-
dollar murder scam.
*Photograph courtesy of the
Glendale Police Department*

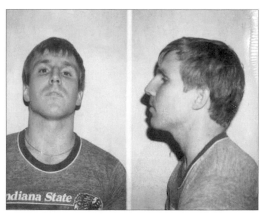

Michael Swango—
already a killer at the time of this 1984 arrest.
Photograph courtesy of the Quincy Police Department

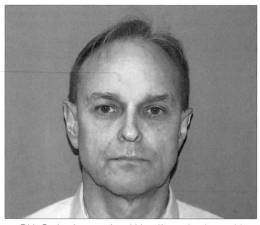

Dirk Greineder—murdered his wife so that he could
satisfy his sexual cravings.
Photograph courtesy of the Wellesley Police Department

met John Branion at Englewood High School, while both were in their teens. High-school sweethearts, they graduated with the class of 1943 and married five years later.

Branion also boasted a strong legal background—his father made history when he was named Illinois's first black assistant public defender—but any hopes that John Jr. would carry on the family tradition were dashed by his decision to opt for medicine as a career. Given his undoubted acumen, he probably would have triumphed in any profession. Branion collected degrees the way other people collect stamps: a masters from the University of Illinois, a Ph.D. in pharmacology, an MD from the University of Lausanne in Switzerland. The excursions abroad also gave him something else, a glossy urbanity rarely found on the Hyde Park dinner party circuit. John and Donna Branion were welcome additions to anyone's guest list, even if the doctor's slick self-preoccupation was at times a little hard to swallow

Close friends knew that beneath Branion's sleek veneer beat a steely resolve. Growing up black in the thirties and forties was tough, no matter how successful your father was or where you lived. Northern-style racial prejudice walked a warier path than the one trod down in Dixie, but hit just as hard. Branion knew that better than most. During the mid-sixties he had taken his lumps in the struggle for civil rights, marching alongside Martin Luther King, Jr., hearing the slurs, braving the taunts and occasional bottles, although whether his motives were solely idealistic is open to dispute. Brushing up against the famous and the powerful meant a lot to Branion. On a few occasions he treated King medically and never missed an opportunity to brag about it afterwards. Branion didn't just bathe in reflected glory, he wallowed in it, littering his conversation with ref-

erences to the shakers and the movers he knew, no matter
how fleetingly.

By 1967 the Branions had reached a comfortable middle age, with two sons, a solid income and as many invitations to social events as they could handle. Acquaintances
knew them as a family to be proud of, hard working, ambitious, happy. As for Dr. John Branion, well, he couldn't
have asked for anything more from his wife. Besides being
a superb mother, Donna was selfless in her devotion to
him. Nothing was too much trouble, not if it helped John
further his career.

Like today.

After finishing the Christmas decorations, Donna
fussed over the guest list for a dinner party she had planned
for that evening. She was a meticulous hostess. Everything
had to be just so.

Meanwhile, the clock moved on to show eleven.

At a few minutes past the hour the woman who lived
next door, Theresa Kentra, came home from a trip to the
grocery store. She hurried in out of the cold, glanced at the
clock and clucked her annoyance—11:05 AM—the shopping trip had taken longer than she'd expected. She began
putting the groceries away. Sometime later, she wasn't sure
exactly when but guessed it was around 11:25 AM, she
heard a loud thud, followed by two or three similar sounds
and a commotion of some sort, all coming from the
Branion residence. She listened further. Nothing. Thinking
no more of it, Theresa Kentra got on with lunch.

Someone else with food on his mind was Dr. John
Branion. Following his daily custom, he left the hospital at
11:30 AM and drove to pick his son up and take him home
for the midday meal. By his own account, when Branion
arrived at the school at 11:35 AM his son was already waiting outside for him. Branion next drove a couple of blocks

to the office of a friend, Maxine Brown. The previous evening Branion had telephoned Mrs. Brown and invited her to lunch the next day with himself and his wife. She had tentatively agreed but, today, when Branion stopped by, Mrs. Brown regretted that, owing to a business commitment, she was unable to keep their lunch engagement. Branion seemed disappointed, pushy almost. Was she sure? "'Fraid so," said Mrs. Brown. Branion shrugged off his dejection and headed home. He arrived at approximately 11:45 AM. In all, from the time he had left Ida Mae Scott Hospital until reaching his home at 5054 South Woodlawn Avenue, John Branion had driven 2.8 miles in rather less than twenty minutes. A strange silence hung over the apartment when Branion arrived. He and his son entered the living room. The Christmas tree smelled fresh and fragrant, already showering pine needles on the presents below. Branion looked about him and frowned. Where was Donna? She should be here. Calling out her name, he looked in the bedroom.

Deserted.

He moved into the kitchen.

Still no one.

Just off the kitchen there was a small utility room which housed the washing machine. Branion tried the door. The room was in darkness. He flicked on the light.

Seconds later Branion fled from the house, shouting, "Helen! Helen!"

The time was 11:57 AM.

"Helen" turned out to be Helen Payne, one of Branion's neighbors, also a doctor. Even before she could arrive, however, the police were on the scene. Officer William Catizone had received word of Branion's emergency call on his patrol-car radio at midday and raced immediately to Woodlawn Avenue. Already, neighbors were beginning to gather outside. Catizone pushed his way through the crowd and entered the house. Branion, weak and frail looking, motioned him to the laundry room.

Catizone peered in and felt his stomach heave. Donna Branion was lying faceup on the floor, head haloed by a spreading pool of blood, arms akimbo, with her legs pressed together and bent slightly to the right. Four large-caliber bullet holes had shredded her head, face and neck. A final, ugly touch—the killer had knotted a cord so tightly around her neck that it was almost buried in the swollen, purple flesh.

When Dr. Helen Payne arrived her examination, brief through necessity not indifference, confirmed the obvious—Donna Brown was beyond medical assistance.

Dr. Payne turned her attention to Branion. He stood like a man in a trance, all the while staring at Donna's body, transfixed, horror-stricken. His hands shook and the only sound he made was a low continuous moan. Attempts at consolation were fruitless. It was as if John Branion had temporarily lost touch with reality.

He remained that way as an army of forensic specialists swarmed through his home, collecting their samples, their photos, their bits of hair, lint, blood and fibers; all the little things that killers leave behind them. They recovered three expended bullets and four cartridge casings. Two of the bullets were under the body and one near it. A fourth, still in the body, was found later during the autopsy.

Detectives did their best to coax a story from the shocked husband. Branion, still dazed, offered robbery as the only motive for anyone wanting to kill his wife. Asked if there was any sign of theft, he made a cursory check of the house and said there was not. He told of walking through the house, calling out several times for his wife, then finding her covered with blood in the laundry room.

His first instinct had been to spare his son such a ghastly sight. He'd run out into the garden, yelling for help, before returning to dial 911.

The police were curious. Had he examined his wife to check whether she was actually dead?

Branion shook his head. He hadn't needed to. She was obviously dead. His trained eye had spotted the lividity in her legs.* Pulses quickened among the investigators. What kind of husband wouldn't try to help his stricken wife?

Again the parallel with the Wallace case is uncanny. Like Wallace before him, Branion was condemned more for what he didn't do than for what he did. A simple act of omission branded him as abnormal; this ignored the fact that reactions to tragedy are as varied as the people who suffer them. (At the time of Julia Wallace's death, husband William attracted immediate suspicion because of his cool demeanor. A little more breast beating—not something William Wallace was known for—might have saved him an immense amount of grief later on.)

That afternoon Branion was taken to the local police station where he offered an account of his movements that morning: the hospital till 11:30 AM, then the school, on to Maxine Brown's house, his own place around 11:45 AM. At first glance, nothing suspicious, but already detectives were beginning to feel uneasy.

First, they needed to establish the time of Donna Branion's death. Theresa Kentra's statement gave them a likely time of around 11:30 AM. Yet another neighbor was able to pinpoint it even more closely. As luck would have it this man had been indoors awaiting a long-distance tele-

---

*Lividity is the tendency of blood to settle in the lower extremities of a corpse. It begins as soon as the heart stops pumping and causes discoloration of the flesh, usually about thirty minutes after death.

phone call from a friend. Scheduled for 11:30 AM, the call had come through right on time.

While talking on the telephone, the neighbor kept one eye on the clock, conscious of the long-distance telephone charges. The hands had just moved to 11:36 AM when he heard what sounded like gunshots. Telling his caller to hold on a moment, he put the phone down and listened intently. There was only silence. Thinking it couldn't have been anything serious, the man continued his conversation. The call lasted until 11:45 AM. After hanging up, the neighbor recounted the highlights of the conversation to his wife for a few minutes, until they were both interrupted by Dr. Branion's frantic cries for assistance.

If this neighbor's version of events was accurate—and there was no reason to doubt him—then Donna Branion had died at the very time when Branion was picking up his son from the nursery school, one mile away. Corroboration came from the telephone company. Their records, showing similar timing almost to the minute, enabled the authorities to eliminate Branion from suspicion.

The mood at police headquarters grew glum. Time is always the criminal's ally; each passing hour makes the chances of an arrest that much more remote. And this case seemed particularly baffffing: no motive, no suspect, no weapon, nothing. But help was on its way, courtesy of the forensic analysts.

The bullets that killed Donna Branion were of .38 caliber; quite common, but microscopic examination revealed very distinctive rifling patterns (grooves and scratches made on the bullet as it travels along the gun barrel). These allowed them positively to identify the murder weapon as a Walther PPK, a rare automatic pistol. Branion, an avid gun collector, was asked if he owned any weapon capable of firing .38 caliber ammunition. He replied only one, a .38

Hi Standard. No mention was made of a Walther PPK. Again, Branion appeared to be in the clear.

And then he did something remarkably stupid.

Just forty-eight hours after the murder of his wife, Dr. John Marshall Branion, bereaved husband and grieving father, hopped on a plane and flew off to Vail, Colorado for a Christmas getaway. First his perceived callousness at the murder scene, now this. Dr. Branion was appearing very much like a man who didn't give a damn about his wife's death, or his kids for that matter. Now it was a question of deciding whether the doctor was just plain insensitive . . . or something worse.

Branion's ill-timed sojourn in the Rockies lit a fire under an otherwise lukewarm investigation. While he lived it up on the slopes of a Colorado ski resort, back in Chicago an increasingly skeptical band of detectives were taking his story apart with an almost surgical precision.

They began making the rounds of the neighborhood, asking questions, jogging memories. Did anyone remember anyone or anything suspicious; something that might shed some light on this seemingly inexplicable murder? While no one came right out and said so, little by little, almost reluctantly, hints were dropped, the sum of which suggested that the Branions' ideal marriage might not be so perfect after all.

What was wrong?

Fights, said the neighbors. Not just everyday spats, like most married couples have on occasion, but real brawls that lasted long into the night, for days on end, filled with the kind of shouting and screaming that was impossible to ignore.

The investigators didn't push this line of questioning, knowing that, eventually, the neighbors would reveal the reason for such discord. Besides, they already had their suspicions. Nine times out of ten when financially secure couples fight like alley cats, they tend to do so for the oldest of reasons. Sure enough, for the past several months Donna Branion had been convinced that her husband was seeing another woman, maybe even more than one. Her highly vocal accusations had been vehemently denied by Branion, though he had been heard to yell back that, if he did seek the comfort of another woman's charms, then the fault would lie with Donna herself.

Confirmation of Branion's infidelity came from many sources. With Donna beginning to show the signs of incipient middle age and, from what neighbors said, an increasing disinterest in marital relations, her husband found no shortage of women willing to take up the sexual slack. By 1967 his libidinous eye had firmly settled on one person, Shirley Hudson, a nurse with whom he worked. From all accounts they were close, very close.

Employing this information, detectives stitched together a reasonable hypothesis of a man at the end of his marital tether, wanting to be free of an unhappy marriage, but fearing the financial ruin that divorce could bring. In such a situation, for such a man, murder might be an attractive proposition. The idea began to form that perhaps Branion had hired someone to kill his wife. Life was cheap on Chicago's South Side, a couple of hundred bucks was enough to get anyone eliminated. But before exploring this possibility, the police decided to look more closely at Branion's movements on the day of the murder.

Nothing arouses official suspicion more than a seemingly cast-iron alibi. In real life it rarely happens. But Branion seemed to have every minute covered. When Detective Michael Boyle drove the route Branion had taken, however, he noticed something interesting—it took him right past Branion's own home. Boyle speculated:

could Branion have murdered his wife, then hurried off to establish an alibi? Given his stated chronology of events it didn't seem possible. But what if the doctor had lied? What if his timings were deliberately off by just a few minutes?

At the hospital Boyle learned that Branion had finished his rounds shortly before 11:30 AM. His last patient, a young man suffering from a minor chest ailment, recalled Dr. Branion coming to his room at 11:25 AM. He remembered the time precisely because, like most hospital patients, he was bored lying in bed and looked forward to the doctor's visit to break the monotony. The patient remarked that Dr. Branion had seemed preoccupied, eager to conclude the visit. After less than a minute the doctor was gone.

Boyle drove to the nursery. He spoke with Mrs. Joyce Kelly, an assistant school supervisor. She reacted angrily when told of Branion's statement that his son was dressed and waiting outside when he had arrived at 11:35 AM. Under no circumstances, she told Boyle angrily, would she allow a four-year-old child to be left outside on a busy thoroughfare to wait for a parent. And on such a bitterly cold day, around 21 degrees! Besides, she sniffed, Boyle was quite wrong in saying that Dr. Branion had arrived at 11:35 AM. She knew very well what time the doctor arrived. She should, since he was fifteen minutes late. He had pulled up at 11:45 AM.

Boyle looked up sharply. He questioned how Mrs. Kelly could be so certain of the time; surely she had other children to look after and could not be expected to log the exact arrival time of each parent? Joyce Kelly agreed, but added that her second class of preschoolers was due at noon and she'd kept watching the clock, worried that hospital duties would detain Dr. Branion. When she saw his car pull up in front of the school, she glanced at the clock and was relieved to note that she had fifteen minutes to tidy up in preparation for her next class.

There was more. Mrs. Kelly had watched Branion race into the school and the day room where his son was waiting. She said he seemed incredibly rushed for time, kneeling down and forcing the little boy into his winter coat and gloves. Once the child was dressed—a matter of a minute or so later—Branion scooped the boy up in his arms and left. Mrs. Kelly, somewhat flustered by all this whirlwind activity, watched the doctor bundle his child into the front passenger seat, then run around to the driver's seat. In a squeal of tires, he made a hurried U-turn and sped off in the direction of his home.

Boyle had plenty to occupy his mind as he left the nursery school. If Mrs. Kelly's recollections were accurate, then at least ten minutes of Branion's journey were unaccounted for. And slap in the middle of those ten minutes was 11:36 AM, the very time when the neighbor on the telephone heard the gunshots that killed Donna Branion.

Next, Boyle interviewed the woman who had arranged to have lunch with the Branions that day. Maxine Brown told essentially the same story as Branion. But she added something Boyle hadn't heard before, something which sounded highly suspicious. The arrangements, she said, had come out of the blue on the night before. She was already in bed when the phone rang at 10:30 PM. It was Dr. Branion, inviting her to lunch the following day with himself and his wife. Maxine Brown had thought the request odd, first of all because Branion had never made such a request before, and also because of the lateness and the gentle but firm insistence on his part that she accept. Mrs. Brown had tentatively agreed, with the proviso that business pressures might necessitate a cancellation. Branion said he would call anyway.

Now the contradictions came thick and fast. The floodgates were open and the tide was running firmly against Branion. When Dr. Helen Payne, who'd examined Donna Branion and pronounced her dead, heard that Branion had not bothered assisting his wife because he had spotted the lividity in her legs, she was stunned. Impossible, she said. She would stake her reputation on the fact that lividity was not present. If Branion claimed otherwise, maintained Dr. Payne, he was mistaken.

Not mistaken, reasoned detectives, lying. They believed that Branion had gone directly from the hospital to his house, killed Donna, then driven to the nursery school to establish his alibi. That was the theory. Now it was necessary to see if it was possible in practice.

In 1931 a team of Liverpool police officers had set out similarly to explode the alibi of William Wallace. They did it by huffing and puffing their way across Liverpool on foot and by tram; these antics caused much amusement among the locals and earned for the seriously out-of-condition officers the derisive nickname the "Anfield Harriers."

Their Chicago counterparts in 1968 had it rather easier. Boyle and a partner were spared any neighborhood scorn. Their test runs of Branion's alleged route, conducted by patrol car, also produced more conclusive results. Over six trips, in a variety of weather and traffic conditions, they covered the 2.8-mile journey in a minimum of six minutes and a maximum of twelve. This was time enough for Branion to have committed the murder and then gone to pick up his son. Damaging as this hypothesis was, Boyle still couldn't uncover any direct evidence to connect Branion with the death of his wife.

In the meantime community frustration found expression in a stinging series of editorials in the *Daily Defender*, Chicago's premier black newspaper. Complaints that the police didn't pursue the murderers of blacks as diligently as those of white victims found a ready audience. In this case it wasn't true, but that was the general perception.

With criticism mounting, the police finally got a break. Walter Hooks, a friend of Branion's, admitted that, in February 1967 (ten months before the shooting), he had given the doctor a belated birthday gift—a Walther PPK automatic, the kind of weapon used to kill Donna Branion.

On January 22, 1968, Boyle returned to Branion's apartment. This time he had a search warrant. He didn't find the gun but, in a cabinet which had been locked on the day of the murder, he found a brochure for a Walther PPK, an extra ammunition clip and a manufacturer's target, all bearing the serial number 188274, the same number as the gun given to Branion by Hooks. He also found two boxes of Geco brand .38 caliber ammunition, recovered from a cupboard in the den. One box was full and contained twenty-five bullets, the other box was missing four bullets, the same number of shots that had killed Donna Branion.

When confronted by these revelations, Branion blustered. Ahhhh . . . now it came back to him. Yes, he remembered the Walther . . . but it must have been stolen by the intruders who killed his wife . . . when they took the $500.

"What $500?" asked Boyle.

"The $500 that was stolen during the robbery."

"Why didn't you mention this money before?" said Boyle.

"I hadn't noticed it missing before."

Not surprisingly, following this exchange, Branion was taken into custody and booked on charges of first degree murder.

• • •

On May 28, 1968, after a two-week trial, eleven white and one black jurors found Dr. John Marshall Branion, Jr. guilty of murder. He was sentenced to twenty to thirty years' imprisonment. The verdict stunned Chicago's South Side. This wasn't the outcome they had expected or wanted. In their eyes Branion, one of the black community's most prominent citizens, had been convicted on the flimsiest of circumstantial evidence and many still believed his story of murderous intruders. Moreover, Branion's lawyer claimed that his client was a victim of the city's recent racial turmoil, making it impossible for him to receive a fair trial. This was a theme that Branion would harp on incessantly, the fact that he was a conspicuous civil-rights activist, tried more for his politics than for any crime.

Trial Judge Reginald J. Holzer was also not enthusiastic about the verdict. He, too, felt that the evidence, although weighty, was not enough to preclude the possibility of a reasonable doubt. Within days word began filtering out from Holzer's chambers, indicating that "Hizzoner" might overturn the verdict. Getting wind of this rumor, prosecutor Patrick Tuite took the decidedly unorthodox step of calling on the judge, urging him to let the Appellate Court decide the outcome. Such conversations, while unethical, were a regular feature of Chicago judicial life at the time and, besides, Tuite knew something else that was also common knowledge in Circuit Court—Judge Holzer was a crook.

Not just any crook, but the biggest crook in a judiciary that could, with some justification, lay claim to being the most corrupt in America. Holzer had been on the take for years. At his peak Judge Holzer managed to spend $100,000 annually and stack up personal debts of

$500,000, all on a judge's salary of $43,500. How he achieved this dubious financial status needs some explanation. First there was his habit of borrowing heavily from lawyers who appeared before him, then conveniently forgetting to pay them back. At other times Holzer made counsel aware that prospects of a favorable ruling from the bench would be greatly enhanced if they placed their insurance business with the judge's wife, Estelle, who ran a thriving agency. Conditioned by the harsh realities of day-to-day Cook County justice, lawyers gritted their teeth and coughed up. That was how the system worked. Or at least it did until 1986. That was when Judge Reginald Holzer was jailed for eighteen years, nabbed by the "Greylord" operation, an FBI sweep that netted dozens of Chicago's less principled legal practitioners.

But all that was in the future. In the summer of 1968 Judge Holzer was still ruling the roost at Circuit Court and, according to rumor, was genuinely upset by Branion's conviction. Never a man to act on conscience alone, Holzer put out a few feelers. For the right price he was prepared to reverse the jury's decision. In an affidavit sworn years later, Nelson Brown, Branion's brother-in-law, claimed to have paid Holzer $10,000, with the promise of $10,000 more if Branion's conviction was overturned. Everything was set.

And then prosecutor Tuite paid his unexpected visit to Holzer's office.

The judge reacted predictably. He pocketed Brown's money and let the conviction stand. But he did do something decidedly odd—he set Branion, a convicted murderer, free on $5,000 bail. It cost the doctor just $500, 10 percent of the bail bond, to get back on the streets.

Barely three months later he married longtime companion Shirley Hudson. Further surprises were in store. In an almost unparalleled example of leniency, doctor and bride were next permitted to move to Cheyenne, Wyoming, while his case meandered along the appellate corridors.

The hiatus lasted three years. In that time Branion saw every court uphold his conviction. By 1971 the appeal process had worked its way through to the Supreme Court. It was a last-ditch effort and Branion knew it. With chances of the conviction being overturned virtually nonexistent, the South Side physician played his trump card.

He disappeared.

It was as though Dr. John Marshall Branion had been wiped from the face of the earth. Friends and relatives of the missing doctor, when questioned by the police, all shook their heads; no one admitted having seen him. A similar response greeted the wanted posters that went to every United States post office. Investigators were certain that it was only a matter of time before they nailed Branion; after all, he couldn't leave the country because his passport had been surrendered at the time of bail. But they had grossly underestimated the doctor's resourcefulness. This was no hasty, spur-of-the-moment decision; every step had been carefully thought out in years of planning.

Even before leaving Chicago, Branion had acquired a new passport, using a ridiculously simple technique. At that time, Uncle Sam checked only birth records before issuing a passport. All Branion had to do was find someone of similar age to himself who had died, then apply for a passport in that person's name. As luck would have it, Arthur McCoo, a friend of Branion's, fit the bill perfectly. Branion wrote to City Hall in Chicago, enclosing the fee and requesting a copy of McCoo's birth certificate. When this arrived he then applied for a driver's license in the dead man's name. With just these two pieces of documentation he was able to obtain a new, perfectly genuine passport in the name of Arthur McCoo.*

Branion bided his time, cognizant of just how tardy the judicial process could be. But with the Supreme Court set to rule, he made his move. From Denver he flew to Boston. At Logan Airport he showed his passport in the name of Arthur McCoo, then boarded a transatlantic flight. One of modern history's most extraordinary man-on-the-run sagas had just begun.

After going to ground in Paris, Branion travelled to Algeria. The destination was perfect for him. He spoke French fluently and Algeria was a place where he could subjugate his American background. Things worked out well. His passport went unchallenged, he was well financed (funds were wired to him from America), and each day boosted his confidence. Not that he needed much of the latter; it was there in reckless abundance. Most fugitives on the run would elect to keep their heads down and hope to avoid publicity. Not Branion. That wasn't his style at all. Algeria restored his old cockiness and, with it, that yearning for the big names and the limelight. The country had its share of both. Eldridge Cleaver, American revolutionary and leader of the Black Panther Party, was frantically trying to drum up support for a halfwitted "invasion" of the United States by the Panthers. Branion was drawn to Cleaver like a moth to a flame but, after a while, began to realize the precariousness of his situation. All that talk of revolution could only draw heat from the CIA and possible discovery. Wisely Branion distanced himself from Cleaver

---

*A word of caution to anyone seeking to employ this strategy nowadays; this loophole has long since been closed!

and set about building a new life. He might have succeeded had fate not intervened—he lost his passport in a taxi.

Branion panicked. Cleaver told him that it was no big deal; he should call at the American Embassy and request a duplicate. Three days later the original passport was returned to Branion by the taxi driver but, by then, he had already gone to the embassy. Worse still, he had created suspicion. During his interview Branion drew a blank on details of McCoo's birthdate and relevant family information. In a funk he made up names and dates on the spot, hoping to bluff his way through. The embassy, deeply suspicious, issued him with a temporary passport only, valid for three months.

Again Branion decamped, this time to Khartoum in the Sudan. Again he was not safe. Word had passed along diplomatic channels of a middle-aged American traveling on false papers. The local US embassy told the Sudanese authorities and had him thrown in jail where he languished for six months until payment of a fine secured his release. Strangely enough, during his incarceration American diplomats apparently made no serious attempt to discover Branion's real identity. (Branion later claimed that these diplomats knew exactly who he was, but chose to ignore it. He offered no reason for their inertia.)

Tanzania was his next stop. Here, he was able to employ his professional qualifications for the first time when a private medical firm in Dar es Salaam hired him as a gynecologist. He earned steady if unspectacular money, enough for him to send for his wife, Shirley, and two sons. They flew in from America and, for a while, life could not have been better. However, familial bliss underwent a severe dislocation when, out of the blue, Branion was summoned before the Tanzanian Immigration Department. There an official stamped his passport "persona non grata" and told him to "get the hell out of the country within two weeks."

After stints in Senegal and the Ivory Coast, Branion was forced to send his family back to America while he continued looking for a country that would grant him refuge. He became a kind of Flying Dutchman, casting around all over the continent for a safe haven. Salvation came in Uganda, then firmly under the iron fist of Africa's dictator-in-chief, President Idi Amin.

Using the alias "John Busingye" Branion was given a hospital post in Mbarara, a small town near Lake Victoria. He thrived and on Amin's personal say-so was granted Ugandan citizenship and a passport. For a while Branion even acted as personal physician to the despot, dismissing as British propaganda reports that Amin's somewhat alarming character defects were prompted by the ravages of advanced syphilis. Later, Branion would become a strident apologist for Amin, excusing his savageries against Indian businessmen with the words, "It was time to kick out the Asians . . . because they had control of the economy . . . no leader should let that kind of thing go on forever."

Life in the latter half of the seventies was good for Branion. At last, it seemed, his running days were over. He had a good job, spacious accommodation, the personal patronage of a powerful dictator and those high-profile social contacts that he doted on. Among his Ugandan acquaintances were radical activist Stokely Carmichael and his wife, singer Miriam Makeba; also Roy Ennis, leader of the New York-based Congress of Racial Equality (CORE). Whether these visitors were aware that the doctor was a convicted killer is unknown. But Branion's luck then became uncertain. This time it was his health. A heart attack forced him to fly to Switzerland for double-bypass surgery.

After a lengthy recuperation, which included big-game fishing in Kenya, he returned to Uganda in 1979. But times had changed. Amin was gone, victim of a coup that banished him into exile. Under new President Milton Obote, Branion's position was never so secure, but he managed to land a teaching job at Makerere University. It lasted long enough for him again to summon his family from America in 1982.

One year later Branion's remarkable odyssey came to a sudden and decisive end. Officially the new regime, learning that he had secured his passport only through the intervention of the hated Amin, declared him "an undesirable immigrant" and ordered his extradition. More likely is that Branion simply ran out of money and could no longer afford to grease the bureaucratic wheels that had kept him out of American custody.

A deportation order delivered him into the hands of two Cook County sheriffs at Entebbe Airport and, on October 15, 1983, bearded and bespectacled, Dr. John Branion was returned to the United States in handcuffs. Twelve years of life on the run was over.

Even behind prison bars Branion continued to rally support around him. Fresh ammunition for his cause came in 1986 when Judge Holzer's racketeering conviction revealed details of the earlier alleged bribe attempt. Branion's lawyers demanded a retrial on grounds that such conduct had denied their client a fair hearing. It was a desperately weak argument. Holzer, whether through genuine doubts or, more likely, avarice, was patently sympathetic to Branion during the trial. How his alleged solicitation of a bribe could be construed as prejudicial towards Branion flies in the face of common sense. The courts agreed. Despite numerous appeals, motions, even pleas on television, Branion remained in prison until August 1990 when he was abruptly freed on health grounds. He had served just seven years of his sentence.

A storm of complaints greeted his release, but Illinois Governor James Thompson had acted in good faith and with great compassion. Branion posed no threat to society, and he was a very sick man. One month later, at the age of sixty-four, he died of a brain tumor and heart trouble.

So was Dr. John Branion an innocent man caught in a web of incriminating circumstances, forced into a life on the run? Or was he a calculating killer, someone who carefully schemed his wife's murder, then fled to escape the consequences? He has no shortage of supporters who believe him wholly innocent. They point to the tainted nature of his trial, the questionable racial tension, Judge Holzer's supposedly improper conduct. But in the final analysis it is difficult to dispute the jury's decision. Branion's roller-coaster alibi had too many holes in it, as did his later statements to the police. At his trial Branion chose not to testify; judging from subsequent events, this was probably a wise decision. In 1988 the ailing doctor presented his side of the story. He did it before the merciless glare of television cameras. For the first time Branion's vanity became a matter of public record. Still adamant in his insistence that Donna had been murdered by intruders, Branion was disdainful of suggestions that he had killed his wife in order more readily to facilitate an illicit liaison. Why, he scoffed, bother to commit murder when he had the best of both worlds—a wife at home, ready to cook and look after him, and a lover elsewhere, eager to accommodate his sexual needs? A man would be insane to ruin such a perfect situation!

Such overweening arrogance damned him more than any evidence. In common with most narcissists, Branion had a rich strain of stupidity running through him, one which entirely misjudged the odium that his performance generated. Hubris-ridden, unremorseful, concerned only with his own predicament, the doctor left few viewers doubting that it was indeed his hand on the gun that had killed Donna Branion all those years before.

9. THE BUSINESS OF MURDER

Paris: March 11, 1944. For days thick columns of greasy black smoke had belched from the chimney of 21 rue le Sueur, an elegant three-story villa set in the capital's fashionable Etoile district. Neighbors eyed the smoke balefully, their noses and stomachs rebelling against its sickening stink. They were used to some strange comings and goings at number 21, most often during the blackout hours, but nothing like this. Finally, Jacques Marcais, who lived opposite, decided enough was enough. He telephoned the police and demanded action.

In war-torn Paris smoky chimneys, no matter how vile, rated low on the list of official priorities, so it was some time before two gendarmes arrived to investigate the complaint. Officers Teyssier and Fillion dismounted from their bicycles, sniffed the air and agreed with Marcais—disgusting.

Pinned to the large, ornate double doors, a note meant for the postman declared that the occupant would be away for a month and gave an address for redelivery. The gendarmes knocked anyway but got no response. After examining the tightly shuttered windows, they went next door and spoke to the concierge. She advised them that the owner of number 21 was a doctor who lived about three kilometers away. She had his telephone number.

The doctor's wife took the call, then summoned her husband. He asked Teyssier quickly, "Have you entered the building?" Told they had not, he added, "Don't do anything. I will be there with the keys in a quarter of an hour."

Thirty minutes passed. Still no doctor. Smoke continued to blacken the sky. Teyssier's patience first stretched, then snapped. He phoned the fire brigade. In minutes a fire truck came clanking along the rue le Sueur. Fire Chief Boudringhin and some of his men scaled the wall, forced an upstairs window and clambered inside. The house was large, fifteen rooms, but they soon tracked the source of the smoke to the basement furnace.

As he led his men into the room, Boudringhin was confronted by a spectacle beyond belief. His eyes widened with horror. Behind him the other firemen could only gape. One had to turn away and retch.

Someone had stuffed the pot-bellied stove full of human corpses.

The floor of this smoke-filled hellhole was also littered with countless body parts—bones, gristle, rotting lumps of flesh, all awaiting despatch in the makeshift crematorium. Whoever had started this barbecue obviously intended that it should last a while.

Ashen-faced and trembling, Boudringhin ran to the front door, threw it open and sucked in welcome mouthfuls of cool, clean March air. He beckoned to the gendarmes, then said with commendable understatement, "Gentlemen, I think you have some work ahead of you."

Just then a middle-aged man, well dressed, short and

stocky with dark unruly hair, came cycling along the street. He slowed down outside number 21. His black eyes glittered when he saw the door ajar. For a moment he considered riding straight past, but bravado got the better of him. He'd fooled them before; he could do it again. Leaning his cycle against the wall, the little fellow stepped inside, confident. After all, if anyone could pull the wool over their eyes, it was Dr. Petiot . . .

His full name was Marcel André Henri Félix Petiot and he was born in 1897, the son of a postal worker in Auxerre, a smallish town some 160 kilometers south of Paris. Right from the cradle, the madness that would shape his extraordinary life shone beacon bright. Most infants are cruel; Petiot was a pure sadist. When he was just five years old a nursemaid caught him dunking a neighbor's kitten in boiling water. The nurse at first scolded young Petiot then, believing he showed some remorse, allowed him to take the kitten to bed with him. The next morning the kitten was stiff as a board; it had been smothered. Petiot innocently disclaimed all knowledge of the episode, but the smirk on his scratched and bloody face said otherwise.

Another favorite nursery pastime was stealing fledglings from their nests, poking out their eyes with a needle, then tossing them into a cage and gloating over their blind, pathetic efforts at escape. As a spectacle it never failed to reduce the young lad to gales of manic laughter.

For Petiot, the commonplaces of the schoolroom were to be challenged rather than accepted. He once interrupted a lesson by firing his father's revolver into the classroom ceiling, then was caught hurling knives, circus style, with unnerving accuracy around a small boy who stood terrified against a door. Such diversions tended to overshadow his undoubted academic brilliance. His memory was phenomenal. In later life he would devour popular novels at the rate of three hundred pages an hour, and afterward be able to recite long extracts verbatim.

In 1914 Petiot had his first brush with the law. He had always been a thief, stealing from his classmates; now he was caught robbing mailboxes, reaching in with a stick that had glue on the end. Before sentencing he was ordered to undergo a psychiatric evaluation, as was customary in French courts. Petiot, glib and cunning as a fox, bamboozled the doctors completely. Their diagnosis of mental disturbance absolved him of responsibility for his actions and gave the court no alternative but to set him free. To accommodate the judiciaire, Petiot attended a Paris school for maladjusted children, graduating with full honors in July 1915.

It was the worst of times to reach manhood in France. On the Western Front his countrymen were being slaughtered by the millions. With a life expectancy that could be measured in weeks or even days, Petiot went off to war. Against all odds he stayed intact until 1917 when a piece of shrapnel smashed his left foot and put him into the hospital. Ever resourceful, Petiot turned disadvantage to profit by stealing drugs from a casualty clearing station, then selling them on the black market to addicts.

For the duration of hostilities Petiot ricocheted between the trenches and the hospital bed. Each return to the front occasioned another breakdown. How much was malingering and how much was genuine is impossible to know. What is certain is that in 1919 he was discharged from the army on a full disability pension.

With the end of the war came the problem of how best to make a living. Unbelievably, Petiot, who had already been certified abnormal by almost every doctor who examined him, decided that a career in medicine was just the ticket. Even more remarkably, he breezed through the curriculum in less than three years, astounding those around him, none of whom could recall ever having seen him study. However he managed it—and there were some who suspected outright fraud—in December 1921 Marcel Petiot graduated from the Faculté de Médecine de Paris a qualified doctor.

In the provincial towns of France, university degrees from Paris were both noteworthy and scarce; this explains the delight and surprise shown by Villeneuve-sur-Yonne's 4,200 inhabitants when Dr. Petiot set up his surgery there. For a young physician eager to make his way in the world, Villeneuve offered distinct promise. The town had only two doctors and they were both advancing in years, as Petiot was quick to point out in a flier he circulated. Part of it read: "Dr. Petiot is young, and only a young doctor can keep up to date on the latest developments . . . Dr. Petiot treats but does not exploit his patients."

He quickly put together a substantial practice, aided in no small part by his reputation as a doctor unconcerned about fees, a trait sure to impress parsimonious French peasants. What his patients did not know was that Petiot had everyone enrolled in the state scheme; this meant that he was reimbursed for every patient, including the ones who had already paid. His greed was boundless. He once summed up his philosophy to an acquaintance: "To succeed in life, one must have a fortune or a powerful position." He would spend the remainder of his days striving to achieve both.

In all likelihood Petiot's genesis as a murderer came in 1926 when he engaged the services of a beautiful housekeeper named Louise Delavau. Before long it became apparent that she was rather more than just domestic help.

For Petiot this was a first; never before had he evidenced any sign of interest in the opposite sex. Unfortunately, as the relationship blossomed, so did Louise's waistline which soon became a prime topic of local gossip and speculation. Suddenly, with rumor peaking, Louise vanished. Petiot proclaimed himself distraught. Louise had just left him, he said. His patients flocked to commiserate. He accepted their sympathy stoically, promising to get over it.

And there the incident might have lain, except that Petiot was unable to keep his mouth shut. His goading of a local gendarme about bungled police attempts to find Louise stimulated a more concerted investigation of her mysterious disappearance. It soon uncovered something sinister. A villager reported seeing Petiot load an ominously heavy trunk into his car. Shortly afterward a similar trunk, hauled from a nearby river, was found to contain the headless corpse of a young female. Speculation ran rampant. Immersion in water made identification an impossibility, however, and, while suspicion lingered, the rumors concerning Louise's disappearance gradually faded. Not that Petiot minded. On the contrary, he seemed oblivious to such trivia. Besides, he had other things on his mind—politics.

From murder suspect to mayoral candidate was quite a jump, and one which Petiot managed without batting an eyelash. An excellent public speaker, amusing and quick-witted, he had the politician's flair of always knowing how best to play on the affections of his audience. Although an overwhelming favorite to gain the seat, Petiot left nothing to chance. At an election eve town hall meeting when both he and his closest rival were scheduled to deliver an address, Petiot spoke first and received a rousing reception. But no sooner had his opponent taken the podium then a power blackout plunged the entire town into darkness. The timing was immaculate. Earlier, Petiot had armed a supporter with a length of copper cable and precise instructions on how to short circuit Villeneuve's electrical supply. While his rival stormed from the hall in an impotent rage, Petiot soaked up the audience applause and the next day romped home in a landslide.

Predictably, he made an unconventional mayor. To start with, there was the town's exchequer; he seemed incapable of distinguishing between it and his own bank account. Hawk-eyed constituents, however, chose to overlook this weakness because Petiot, for all his foibles, definitely had the knack of getting things done. He lobbied tirelessly for state-aided improvements, installed a new sewer system, brought the elementary school up to date. His crowning mayoral achievement came in a typically bizarre fashion. For months he had urged the railway company to schedule more train stops at Villeneuve. Tired of their rebuffs, Petiot brought attention to the problem by flinging himself from the Paris express while it raced full tilt through Villeneuve. Miraculously he was uninjured, but the stunt captured public imagination, made Petiot a hero and shamed the railway company into making more frequent halts.

With his political star in ascendance, Petiot began eyeing higher office. First, though, he needed a wife. With his customary thoroughness he compiled a list of suitable candidates. Georgette Lablais, daughter of an influential local landowner, not unattractive and wonderfully timid, fit the bill perfectly, and in June 1927 the couple married. Ten months later their only child, Gerhardt, was born.

The change in marital status did nothing to change Petiot. He continued plundering the town's coffers, and the kleptomania that had simmered inside him since childhood now became a regular feature of town life. Each time Petiot visited a friend's house he would pilfer some item;

the next day his wife would discreetly return it. Locals became used to, and tolerated, this quirk. But by 1930 Villeneuve was humming with rumors of something far more sinister about its mayor than mere sticky fingers.

On a March evening, dairy owner Armand Debauve returned home to find his house engulfed in flames. Fighting his way into the kitchen he stumbled over the battered, lifeless body of his wife, Henriette. Police suspected that the killer was probably someone local because this was the night in the month when Debauve always had the most money in his house, almost F250,000. As it happened, the murderer missed this sizeable cache, hidden under a kitchen counter, but he did rifle the safe and steal F20,000.

The discovery of footprints leading toward a nearby stream only reinforced police suspicions that the killer had local knowledge. This was difficult terrain to negotiate in the dark for anyone, for a stranger it would be next to impossible. Later, when gendarmes dragged the stream, they uncovered a hammer that matched exactly the wounds in Henriette's head, but rust and sludge had obliterated any fingerprints or traces of blood.

As days meandered by without an arrest, an unusual series of articles began appearing in a local newspaper. Besides mocking the police for their lack of results, the articles viciously impugned Henriette Debauve's character, suggesting that her morals were less than wholesome, and also predicting that her murder would remain unsolved.

Police efforts to locate the author of these scandalous outbursts turned up an immediate suspect—none other than Mayor Petiot. Astonishment hardened into outright suspicion when one article revealed specific details of the wounds to Henriette's head, information that the police had guarded closely. How, they speculated, had the mayor come by such knowledge?

Also pointing the finger of suspicion at Petiot was a Monsieur Fiscot, who claimed to have seen Petiot outside the Debauve residence at the time of the fire. Moreover, he alleged that Henriette Debauve had been Petiot's mistress, an idea which had already gained some currency about town.

It so happened that Fiscot, like most citizens of Villeneuve, was also Petiot's patient—the doctor had treated him for rheumatism. Now, by the happiest of coincidences, Petiot chose this moment to call on Fiscot and tell him of a miraculous new drug which had just come on the market. Fiscot incautiously hobbled along to Petiot's surgery and received a shot of the "wonder drug." Three hours later he was dead. According to the doctor who examined the corpse, Fiscot died from natural causes. A death certificate and burial authorization followed in close order. Unfortunately the doctor who performed all these tasks was Petiot himself. With their star witness dead, the authorities, reluctant to ruffle Mayor Petiot's feathers unduly, quietly decided to let the matter drop.

Even a scare like this left Petiot unaffected. His larceny continued until 1931 when he was finally caught embezzling town funds and thrown out of office. At the urging of his many supporters he ran again but was defeated in a close contest. Not that it mattered. Craftily, Petiot had hedged his political bets, campaigning for and winning the state post of general councillor. He remained in this more powerful position for only a year, until being suspended from the legislature for tapping electricity from the local electricity company. Reluctantly, the ex-mayor decided it was time to sever connections with Villeneuve and, in

January 1933, Petiot, his wife and son, packed their bags and headed for Paris.

He settled at 66 rue Caumartin and, showing the same drive that had marked his arrival in Villeneuve, soon amassed a panel of more than three thousand devoted patients.* Despite his success, Petiot was incapable of staying honest. This time the rumors were about drugs. In 1935 a woman complained to the police about the baffling death of her daughter who had gone to Petiot to have an abscess lanced. For some reason she had not recovered consciousness after the anaesthetic. The coroner became suspicious and refused to issue a burial certificate. An autopsy revealed significant amounts of morphine but not enough to suggest foul play. Once again Dr. Petiot dodged the ax.

In 1936 he was caught stealing from a bookshop. At his trial Petiot pleaded intermittent insanity and pointed to his army discharge papers as proof. It worked. Acquitted but ordered to undergo psychiatric treatment, after a fortnight Petiot had the psychiatrist eating out of his hand; he convinced the doctor to declare that he was now sane and eligible for release. When a medical commission examined Petiot, they agreed on three points: he was rotten to the core; he had been feigning insanity; and legally he could not be held in custody a minute longer. Petiot left the mental institution in triumph, although the medical commission did gain one small victory; they had a clause inserted into Petiot's police record, highlighting his selective use of the insanity plea. Thereafter Petiot never used this defense again.

---

*Some idea of their loyalty can be gauged from the fact that, years later when things were at their blackest for Petiot, the police had the greatest difficulty in finding any patient who would say a bad word against him.

The next few years saw Petiot prosper enormously. He even managed to avoid the law, except for a running battle with the taxman, who slapped him with ever-increasing demands. After much whining Petiot reluctantly coughed up the excess. It was money desperately needed by the French exchequer . . . the Second World War had just broken out.

With the collapse of Daladier's government and the subsequent Nazi occupation, Paris was plunged into chaos. Strict rationing kept everything in short supply: food, clothing, medicine. Although the entire population was affected, one sector more discommoded than most was the capital's large drug-addict colony. Before the war they had bought their fixes from black-market dealers; now those same dealers were making fortunes in petrol and nylons. For most junkies this meant finding a doctor willing to bend the rules: someone like Marcel Petiot.

He didn't disappoint. His practice included no less than ninety-five registered addicts, well above average. Typically he found a way to profit from the situation. Medical guidelines dictated that an addict should be weaned off drugs by ever-diminishing doses. This Petiot did, but without ever reducing the amount of the prescriptions. Inevitably the excess drugs found their way to the black market. When arrested for this abuse, Petiot received a one-year suspended sentence and F10,000 fine.

All this was a drop in the ocean for someone of Petiot's means. With his practice, his drug-dealing and a lucrative sideline in hard-to-get wartime abortions, he was raking in millions. He plowed much of that cash into property, one building in particular. Situated near the Arc de Triomphe and complete with stables and a courtyard, it had formerly belonged to royalty and Cécile Sorel, a celebrated French actress. Petiot paid F500,000 for the nineteenth-century building, then hired a firm of contractors to undertake major alterations. Oddest of these was the construction of a triangular, windowless room next to the garage. It wasn't large, only eight feet along its longest side, but set into one wall were several heavy iron rings. In the opposite wall, some six feet above the floor, a spyhole peered in. Petiot allayed the builders' curiosity by saying that he intended the house to be a clinic after the war, with this room set aside for scientific experiments. To deter prying neighbors he also had the courtyard wall increased by three feet in height.

Although Petiot rarely used the house—he continued to see patients at his home on rue Caumartin—21 rue le Sueur would soon become the most notorious residence in all France, a testament to the bottomless depths of one man's depravity as he sought to corner the market in mass murder for profit.

The scheme that Petiot evolved was fiendishly simple. Passing himself off as the head of an underground escape network called "Fly-Tox," he let it be known that, for a fee, he could arrange the safe departure of anyone wishing to leave France. With Paris humming over rumors of the death camps to the east, there was no shortage of patrons, mainly Jews, frantic for any means possible to escape the yoke of Nazi tyranny.

Petiot recruited an army of cutthroats to scour the bars, cafés and bistros for potential customers. On the first interview the would-be escapee was told to report to such and such a place with a minimum of luggage, any valuables they might want to take with them and a fee of $2,000. On no account were they to tell anyone. At the second meeting the traveler was met by Petiot himself, glib and smiling, plausibility personified. And who better to trust than a doctor?

One of the first victims of this slick operation was a Polish furrier named Joachim Guschinov. For F25,000 Petiot promised to provide an Argentinian passport and safe passage to South America. Guschinov sold his business and withdrew F2,000,000 from the bank. In January 1942 he stepped inside 21 rue le Sueur and never left. When, a few weeks later, Guschinov's anxious wife inquired about her husband's whereabouts, Petiot produced letters purportedly written by Guschinov from his sanctuary abroad. But the letters were all forged and neither she nor anyone else ever heard from Joachim Guschinov again.

As the operation's efficiency grew, so did the numbers that Petiot was prepared to deal with. Whole families were despatched to their doom. Each time Petiot pocketed not only the fee charged but also his victims' entire savings, their luggage and their clothes; it was a truly integrated murder factory.

How Petiot actually killed his victims remains a matter of speculation. One theory has him injecting the hapless travelers with poison under the guise of administering an antityphoid inoculation; others opt for gassing in the triangular room. Given the room's singular construction, this seems the most likely. At his trial it was suggested that Petiot liked to gloat over the final agonies of his victims through the spyhole. Recalling his childhood sadism towards animals, it doesn't require any great leap of the imagination to accept this as close to the truth.

The sheer scope of Petiot's operation made it inevitable that news of this human traffic would reach the wrong ears and, in 1943, rumors began filtering into Gestapo headquarters about a ring able to transport Jews out of France. It took the secret police no time to track down the minions, but the leader, a shadowy figure known only as "Doctor Eugène," proved annoyingly elusive. To alleviate this frustration, Gestapo officers hit on a typically diabolical solution to their problem.

They approached the wife of Yvan Dreyfus, a Jew awaiting deportation to a concentration camp, with word that they were prepared to release her husband if he would contact "Fly-Tox" and pretend to be a fugitive seeking refuge abroad. Mrs. Dreyfus quickly agreed. Then the Gestapo officer added a demand for F1,000,000. Mrs. Dreyfus drew out every franc she had and handed it over. As promised, Yvan Dreyfus shuffled through the prison gates and into his wife's arms. Their reunion was glorious but brief as Dreyfus had to fulfill his side of the bargain. On May 21, 1943, he was put in touch with the "Fly-Tox" network. Like all the others, Yvan Dreyfus vanished into the ether, but he did lead Gestapo officers straight to the door of Dr. Marcel Petiot.

He was immediately hauled off to jail, charged with having spirited Dreyfus out of the country. Not once, it seems, did the Gestapo ever consider that Petiot was simply murdering these people and pocketing their belongings. They saw only a saboteur, aiding enemies of the state.

Incarceration held no terrors for Petiot. Neither did torture. What he endured at the hands of his jailers at Fresnes Prison would have broken most men, but not the little doctor from Auxerre. To loosen his tongue, Gestapo interrogators dug deep into their repertoire of persuasion techniques. They began with a simple beating, then proceeded to immersion in freezing water until the point of drowning. When that failed, iron bands were clamped around Petiot's head and screwed so tight that his eyes almost bulged from their sockets. Next, his teeth were filed down to the nerves. He spat blood nonstop and yet steadfastly refused to admit anything. His stoicism astounded cellmates, as did the contempt he heaped on his jailers, taunting and deriding them nonstop. It was an incredible bravura performance.

Or was it?

In January 1944, after eight months of fruitless torture, Petiot was abruptly released. Observers have long pondered why the Gestapo did not execute him and have done with it. One theory put forward maintains that Nazi secret police officers *did* unlock the secret of rue le Sueur and, because most of the homicidal doctor's victims were Jews, chose to turn a blind eye in return for a share of the proceeds. As events unfolded this theory seems increasingly feasible.

For whatever reason Petiot left prison, his health in shreds. He limped back to his hometown of Auxerre to recuperate. Like almost everything else about Marcel Petiot, his recovery rate was unbelievable for, within a fortnight, he had returned to Paris and business as usual, killing indiscriminately.

Barely two months later an irate citizen phoned a complaint to the police. Something about a smoky chimney . . .

Petiot breezed into 21 rue le Sueur. Far from being unnerved by the discovery of so many bones and bodies, he first announced that he was the householder's brother, then asked the gendarmes bombastically, "Are you both Frenchmen?" Assured that they were, Petiot went on: "These bodies you have seen are those of Germans and traitors to our country . . . I assume that you have already notified your superiors and that the Germans will soon learn of your discovery. I am the head of a Resistance group and I have three hundred files at my home which must be destroyed before the enemy finds them." Petiot continued this high-handed lecture for some time, brow-beating the gendarmes into feeling guilty for having stumbled into a Resistance execution chamber and possibly jeopardizing the lives of patriots.

As a ploy it was brilliant. The two gendarmes took in the carnage around them and assumed that only something along the lines that Petiot had described could possibly account for this hellish scenario. They told Petiot to hurry on his way before their superiors arrived. Bidding them *au revoir*, Petiot calmly mounted his bicycle and rode off into the night.

He was only just in time. News of the discovery had already reached Gestapo HQ, prompting a hasty telegram to 21 rue le Sueur: "Order From German Authorities. Arrest Petiot. Dangerous Lunatic."

Ironically, this communication was all that the local gendarmerie needed to convince them of Petiot's truthfulness. For the Gestapo to intervene in civilian matters, even murder, was unheard of.* In the light of this command the French investigators deliberately dawdled. When they finally went to interview Petiot at rue Caumartin, they found him gone.

In the meantime pathologists continued to sift through the gruesome remains at 21 rue le Sueur. They had plenty to occupy their time. The house was a scrapyard of human viscera. Bleached bones and half-consumed lumps of flesh poked out of a quicklime pit in the garage. On a stairway leading down to the courtyard, they found a canvas sack containing the headless, left side of a human. It had been split down the middle, like a chicken ready for roasting. And everywhere there were bones: thirty-four recogniza-

---

*Later, this telegram would be held up as proof that the Gestapo had been privy to Petiot's murderous exploits all along.

ble limbs, another thirty-three pounds of charred remains. Despite the seemingly random slaughter, doctors detected signs of definite anatomical knowledge in the dissection. And there was something else . . .

They had seen this handiwork before. In 1942 and 1943 a dozen mutilated bodies had been fished out of the River Seine. The murderer had almost been caught one night, tossing a human hand off a bridge while a barge passed below, but he had vanished into the blackout. The bodies at rue le Sueur showed similar signs of dissection, leading to the inevitable conclusion that one person had been responsible for both series of murders.

Finally convinced that they were dealing with a madman, the civilian police intensified their search. They tracked Petiot to his brother's radio shop in Auxerre. There they found Petiot's wife, Georgette. She disclaimed all knowledge of her husband's activities other than her view that he was connected with the Resistance. But it was Auxerre that yielded the most chilling discovery yet. At a house owned by Petiot's brother, detectives found no less than forty-nine suitcases and bags, all stuffed with clothes and personal belongings, including twenty-nine suits, seventy-nine dresses, five fur coats and sixty-six pairs of shoes.

The police had never seen anything like it, a murderous Aladdin's cave of relics and shattered dreams. Not content with killing and robbing his victims, Petiot clearly intended to sell the clothes off their backs as well. The Auxerre discovery only redoubled efforts to capture Petiot. Even the Gestapo ran columns about the chase in the collaborationist press. But by the end of April the elusive doctor had still not been found and gradually interest faded. One month later he was entirely banished from the headlines. The newspapers had far more momentous news to report—Allied troops had stormed the beaches of Normandy.

The D-Day landings swamped everything else. As the Allies pushed inexorably towards Paris, smashing aside Germany's faltering war machine, the exploits of a lone, mad killer seemed small beer indeed. On August 25, 1944, four years of miserable occupation came to an end when French forces finally liberated the capital. But amid the triumph came recriminations. It was a time for settling old scores. Collaborators were hunted down mercilessly and the quest for justice was turned into a purge. Between 30-40,000 French people were summarily executed by a variety of courts with varying degrees of legality. Many were innocent victims, caught up in the vengeful madness.

With this thirst for retribution came a revival of newspaper interest in Dr. Petiot. Speculation ran high that France's worst-ever murderer was already dead. Reports had his body being pulled from various rivers all over the country. Others claimed that he was now a doctor in one of Hitler's concentration camps, an idea that gained popularity when a spurious confession by an alleged acquaintance was published, painting Petiot in the blackest light possible and calling him a German agent. Most of the article was manifest rubbish, but it did have one beneficial side effect—it flushed the mad doctor out of hiding.

Petiot angrily wrote to a newspaper, *La Resistance*, declaring that he had been framed by the Gestapo which had used his house as a dumping ground for corpses while he was in prison. The Gestapo had created such an uproar about the bodies, he said, to deflect attention from the crushing defeats Germany was suffering at the hands of the Russians in the east. Writing about himself in the third person singular, Petiot, claiming to be an officer in the

Resistance, boasted: "He is doing all he can for the cause . . . Having lost everything but his life, he is self-lessly risking even that under an assumed name . . . forget the filthy Kraut lies that it takes about two grains of good French common sense to see through."

In time the authorities would crow that they captured Petiot by checking this letter's handwriting against every known member of the Free French Forces (FFF); they were thus able to identify the author as a Captain Henri Valéri, who had been a FFF officer for just six weeks. It all sounded rather clever but does not have the benefit of being truthful.

Well before the handwriting results were in, Petiot was under arrest, caught on October 31, 1944 as he left the métro station at Saint Mandé Tourelles in the eastern out-skirts of Paris. Quite how the police learned of his where-abouts remains shrouded in mystery. The arresting officer, a Captain Simonin, who abruptly disappeared, was later revealed to be a notorious collaborator responsible for the execution of dozens of patriots. Thus, the possibility exists that Petiot was undone by a German agent eager to embar-rass the fledgling French government.

Petiot had thrown off his pursuers by the simple expe-dient of growing a beard. With it he looked radically dif-ferent. When captured he had in his possession several different sets of identity papers. As "Captain Valéri" he was under orders assigning him to French Indochina: an-other few weeks and he might have disappeared forever.

He had gone into hiding at a friend's apartment in the rue Fauberg St. Denis. The friend, a housepainter named Georges Redoute, denied all knowledge of the furor sur-rounding Petiot; later, he admitted that Petiot had men-tioned bodies in rue le Sueur, telling him that they were all Germans. Petiot's eccentricity hadn't deserted him in hiding. His habit of posing bare chested at the window had aroused the ire of neighbors and brought him the nickname Tarzan. It had also prompted a complaint to the police.

He was taken to the Quai des Orfèvres. FFF records showed that he had joined on September 27, 1944; he had been given the task of interrogating prisoners. His secretary described him as a gentle man on the whole, but with some curious sadistic traits.

Petiot cheerfully admitted killing all the victims found at rue le Sueur—indeed, he increased the police total to sixty-three—but, he said, they were all either German soldiers or else traitors. This would form the bedrock of his defense, that he was an executioner for the Resistance and that he also helped many Frenchmen to escape. To bolster his claim he named several underground leaders as close colleagues. Unfortunately, all were dead.

Once he was under lock and key the press largely ignored Petiot, as France struggled to rebuild itself after years of Nazi domination. Languishing in Santé Prison awaiting trial, Petiot lapsed into a sulky torpor. He wrote a rambling book, devoted to various gambling systems and ways to beat casinos. Interspersed with these instructions were anecdotes and comments on his Resistance experiences and some general thoughts on philosophy.

Petiot's pretrial incarceration, which lasted over a year, was highlighted by his point-blank refusal to answer any questions about his crimes. His reply to each and every inquiry was "I wish to explain myself in court." Shrewdly, he took advantage of this hiatus to secure the services of the country's top criminal lawyer, René Floriot. Other than that, Petiot sat in his cell all day long reading newspapers or else solving crossword puzzles. His only other indulgence was a newfound passion for cigarettes: he smoked incessantly.

As his trial date drew near, Petiot shook off his lassitude and began to exude an air of expectancy, telling prison guards that it would be a great trial, with himself, of course, both brilliant and amusing by turns. He promised he would make everyone laugh.

To the impartial observer, French criminal trials are ramshackle, chaotic affairs. A three-man panel of judges not only presides over court business but also assists in the jury deliberations. Often, the main judge, or tribunal president, assumes the mantle of official prosecutor, engaging in the kind of pugnacious and, at times, vituperative questioning that would earn their British and American counterparts an immediate and permanent disbarment. The most astonishing thing is that this overwrought system actually works quite well. From among the hysterics and heartfelt angst an occasional grain of truth is sifted, leading on to the next fact, until eventually a satisfactory outcome is achieved.

For someone like Petiot, it provided a one in a million chance to show off his manic brilliance before the entire population. He managed to turn what were already loose proceedings into a carnival. He posed for the cameras, drew caricatures of the judges, cursed witnesses and counsel alike, dozed off and generally acted the fool. At times his comments were inspired but, for the most part, he came off as boorish and petulant, undisguisedly contemptuous of everyone present.

His trial opened at the Palais de Justice on March 18, 1946. By this time some degree of normality had returned to France and Marcel Petiot was once again front-page news. When the charge was read, he stood indicted on twenty-seven counts of murder; no one in the nation's long history had ever faced such a charge. At the trial's commencement, as is customary under French law, the tribunal president read out a lengthy biography cum character assessment of the accused. During its reading Petiot was constantly on his feet, pointing out real and imagined inaccuracies.

President: "He was a mediocre student."

Petiot: "I only got 'very good' on my thesis."

President: "You were well thought of as a doctor. Your patients found you quite seductive."

Petiot: "Why, thank you."

President: "Nonetheless, a woman in the town, Madame Mongin, had several complaints about you, among them that you stole items from her house."

Petiot: "Madame Mongin wanted me to sleep with her. I declined this honor. She lied."

President: "Next you are going to tell me the whole dossier is false."

Petiot: "I wouldn't say that. Only eight tenths of it is false."

At one point Petiot sulked. "I don't care to be treated like a criminal," a strange comment indeed from someone in imminent danger of losing his head.

One of the prosecutors, Pierre Veron, had also been a prominent Resistance officer, and it was he who grilled Petiot on his alleged involvement with the underground movement, firing off a salvo of questions that shattered the core of Petiot's defense.

Veron: "How do you transport plastic explosives?"

Petiot: "Wait a minute, it's coming back to me. Several comrades filled suitcases with plastic explosives and detonated them with a bomb with a timer . . ."

Veron: "What is a 'bomb with a timer'?"

Petiot: "A German grenade . . . you know . . . the ones with the handle. We heard the explosion thirty minutes later . . ."

Veron: "German fragmentation grenades have a seven-second fuse."

Petiot blustered but he had been caught out in an obvious lie. Later in the exchange matters became a little tense when Veron threatened to knock the defendant's teeth in!

Thus, on the first day, was set the tone for all sixteen days to come. The sheer enormity of Petiot's crimes and his outrageous braggadocio at times made the proceedings difficult to follow, but there was one factor he couldn't ignore. Court attendants had covered an entire wall with a mountain of luggage recovered from Auxerre. Those silent cases spoke with a greater eloquence than any prosecution witness. As a stream of relatives testified of loved ones who had contacted Petiot, only to vanish, inexorably their tear-filled eyes were drawn toward the dismal pile.

Petiot's reaction was vicious and predictable. He denounced all the missing relatives as traitors; France should honor him for having rid them of such a blight. Those that he couldn't dismiss as traitors were now abroad in South America. If they chose not to contact their family in France, that was hardly his fault! Petiot's indifference to the mood of the court is hard to fathom. There was no attempt to gain sympathy or converts to his cause. He regarded this entire proceeding as a monumental waste of time. More than anything else, he appeared bored.

On day five of the trial the entire court went to 21 rue le Sueur. They saw the triangular room. They peered through the spyhole. They also visited the cellar off the courtyard which Petiot had filled with lime for "whitewashing" the house. They saw everything, and then they returned to the court and saw that silent pile of luggage. Only Petiot seemed indifferent. He remained vain, arrogant, self-absorbed, wholly malevolent.

As the trial neared its climax, interest reached a fever

pitch. Court passes fetched a fortune on the black market as spectators, many with opera glasses, jammed the public gallery, eager for a glimpse of one of history's most extraordinary killers. Finally, at 9:30 PM April 4, 1946, the seven-member jury and three judges retired to consider their verdict. Because of the trial's complexity, it was expected that reaching a decision might take days. Actually they were back just after midnight. Petiot had filled in the time by signing autographs for anyone who wanted them. He leaned forward to hear the verdict.

Twenty-six times the jury declared him guilty. Amid the pandemonium Petiot was the only one unaffected. Insouciantly he listened as sentence of death was pronounced. His only reaction came on leaving the court. Turning to the howling crowd, he yelled, "I must be avenged," before warders dragged him away.

Following the rejection of his appeal, Petiot waited stoically for the inevitable. Uniquely, condemned prisoners in France were never told the date of their execution until 6:00 PM the evening before, in the belief that this minimized suffering. Further delaying Petiot's date with the guillotine was the official executioner, a man in his late sixties, who decided that this was the ideal time to strike for higher wages. After considerable haggling, he reached agreement with his employers and France's first postwar execution by guillotine was set.

With all the formalities taken care of, French justice moved swiftly. Just forty-eight hours after the dismissal of his appeal, on May 25, 1946, Petiot was awoken from a sound sleep at 4:30 AM and told that his time had come. He dressed slowly, changing from prison garb into the suit he had worn at his trial. He declined the traditional glass of rum and sat quietly smoking while his neck was shaved. His request to use the toilet was denied, prompting him sardonically to observe that, when one went on a long voyage, one took all one's luggage.

Then he was led out into the prison courtyard.

As recently as 1939 France had still conducted executions in public but, following unruly crowd behavior at the guillotining of mass killer Eugene Wiedmann, it was decided that some things are best kept from public view. It is unlikely that Petiot would have cared either way. The prison doctor, a veteran of hundreds of executions, wrote,

> For the first time in my life I saw a man leaving death row, if not dancing, at least showing perfect calm. Most people about to be executed do their best to be courageous, but one senses that it is a stiff and forced courage. Petiot moved with ease, as though he were walking into his office for a routine appointment.

In the shadow of the guillotine Petiot nodded a laconic greeting to the executioner who bound his feet and strapped him to the tilting wooden board. Petiot glanced across at the witnesses. "Gentlemen," he said, "I ask you not to look. This will not be very pretty."

A second later, at 5:05 AM, the table was pivoted into position and the blade flashed down. At least one witness did not heed Petiot's advice. He swore that, at the very moment Petiot's head left his shoulders, the little doctor was actually chuckling.

10. BLOOD AND BLUNDER

In the eyes of most laymen, doctors have at their fingertips any number of devious ways to extinguish life, should they so desire. A quick jab with the hypodermic, some untraceable poison or an embolism-causing bubble of air, and it is all over. Fortunately, two factors conspire to dispel this myth. In the first place, given the extraordinary advances of modern-day forensic science, untraceable murder is nowhere near as easy to accomplish as the mystery novelist would have you believe; secondly, medical murderers, in common with the overwhelming majority of other killers, tend to be remarkably stupid. (I realize, of course, that I may be doing a grave disservice to those practitioners who have successfully employed the tools of their trade to kill and then avoided detection, but one must retain the hope that such deviants are thin on the ground.)

Having said that, however, it is difficult to escape the conclusion that, when Los Angeles surgeon Dr. Bernard Finch embarked on a mission to eliminate his wife, he set new standards for dim-witted devilry. Rarely, if ever, has

murder been so ill conceived, ill executed or ill concealed.
Were it not for the tragic outcome, his bungling efforts
would rank as farce of the highest order. At times, during a
trial bloated with lurid tales of adultery, avarice and more
than its quota of black comedy, it was often easy to lose
sight of the fact that willful murder had been done, that a
woman lay dead, gunned down from behind by a .38 caliber bullet. Just how that bullet came to be fired was a saga
that held America spellbound for almost two years as a trio
of juries wrestled with the question of whether "The
Doctor and the Redhead" were heartless killers or innocent
dupes.

At age forty-two, Dr. Raymond Bernard Finch was lean,
tan, tall and handsome, a gleaming shrine to aerobic excel-
lence. His physical well-being owed much to long hours
on the tennis court—a game at which he excelled—beneath California's benevolent sun. He had the constitution
and stamina of a man half his age, which, considering his
fondness for teenage redheads, was perhaps just as well.
He smiled easily and often. "Call me Bernie," he'd grin to
new acquaintances. Most did, men and women alike, all
bowled over by his unfailing charm.

His financial fitness, too, was equally obvious. Together
with his brother-in-law and several other doctors, Finch
owned and operated the West Covina Medical Center, a
thriving Los Angeles clinic that catered mainly to rich patients. It was an involvement that afforded Finch and his
wife, Barbara, the rarefied kind of lifestyle that dreams
were made of—a one-story, mustard-colored, ranch-style
house nestled in the hills high above the twinkling lights of
Los Angeles; membership of the exclusive South Hills
Country Club; a Cadillac for him, a Chrysler for her.
Professionally, too, he was well considered; confident of

his diagnoses, quick and certain at the operating table, very soothing when it came to his bedside manner. Life had apparently dealt the best of all possible hands to Bernard Finch. Everything he touched turned, if not to gold, then to a very acceptable shade of silver.

Until 1959.

It was in the early part of that year that the world Dr. Bernard Finch had so carefully built first teetered, then threatened to collapse in ruins as everything he held most dear was threatened by the divorce courts. Given the prevailing circumstances, any sensible spouse would have cut his losses and run. Finch should have. But he was vindictive and he was vengeful. Worst of all, he was greedy.

The eight-year marriage to Barbara, that had begun so well, was now in shreds. To hear Finch tell it, the root cause of its failure was her frigidity. Like many ambitious and driven men Finch had a prodigious sexual appetite. Barbara did not. It hadn't always been that way. Ironically, it had been her eager accommodation of his lusty advances which provided the legal ammunition that enabled both to escape from unhappy first marriages and to tie the knot. Barbara brought to the union her daughter, Patti. Finch brought money, undeniable comfort and the promise of a seemingly limitless future. In 1953 the arrival of Raymond Jr. served to cement their relationship and, for a while, life at 2740 Lark Hill Drive took on an idyllic sweep.

But that was then. As the years came and went, Barbara changed. Or so Finch claimed. Now she rejected his every sexual advance. Out of this impasse grew a so-called "open marriage"—more his idea than hers—in which each was free to follow his or her own inclinations. For Finch this meant untrammelled sexual conquest. Barbara settled for an uninterrupted diet of cocktail parties, fundraisers, barbecues, shopping and all the other things that upper-middle-class American housewives were supposed to do in the fifties. So long as Finch did nothing openly to embarrass her, she remained indifferent to him.

At first this arrangement worked well. Finch limited his indiscretions to fleeting trysts with bored housewives—either speedy couplings in parked cars or the occasional jaunt to San Francisco—plus an endless succession of starry-eyed nurses. But in late 1956 something happened that would slam the door shut on this open marriage, changing three individual lives forever, none for the better.

Carole Pappa was eighteen when she first went to work as a secretary at the West Covina Medical Center. Initially she paid little heed to the handsome Dr. Finch—his reputation as a rake was legendary—besides which, she had only been married a month. Husband James was a body freak who laid bricks for a living and pumped iron for fun. Every spare hour was spent in the gym, toning his frame to rippling perfection. Jimmy Pappa's passion for physique possibly explained his devotion to Carole. Her face and figure were breathtaking. Above average in height, with a halo of rich auburn hair framing her perfectly oval face, she had posed for pin-up photos and modeled lingerie until Jimmy put his foot down—he didn't want any other men ogling what he considered to be his and his alone. (It speaks volumes for her startling beauty that, when she later appeared in court, not even the frumpish dress code that defense counsel inevitably imposes on attractive female clients could disguise the fact that Carole Pappa was a knockout.)

The attraction was not lost on Dr. Finch. After seven months as a receptionist, Carole became his personal secretary. If her later account is to be believed, another seven months passed before she yielded to the doctor's persistent attentions. In February 1957 the couple shared a very agreeable hour or two over lunch. Later that week they met for dinner. As Finch gazed into Carole's liquid brown eyes, all sense of time evaporated. They murmured long into the night. When Carole arrived home the clock showed 4:15 AM. Jimmy Pappa was waiting and not amused. All hell broke loose, so badly, in fact, that Carole swore off all forms of sexual contact with her husband. From that night forth she was Finch's alone.

There is little doubt that Finch went overboard for his secretary. In the past his extramarital dalliances had been hasty and furtive, now he threw caution to the winds and, at a cost of $70 per month, rented a small furnished apartment in Monterey Park, five miles from his home. Finch later claimed that Barbara, if not privy to all the details, was certainly aware of, and tolerated, the liaison. It is difficult to imagine how she could have done otherwise since, according to Finch, he and Carole frequented this apartment, and another to which they moved soon afterward, at every available opportunity—lunchtimes, mid-mornings, afternoons and evenings as well. When recalling this period in court later, Finch mixed wistfulness with arrogance as he proudly detailed their sexual encounters in the earthiest of terms. Carole, by contrast, remained stone-faced behind horn-rimmed spectacles, obviously preferring to forget the whole sordid affair.

But for now they were in love and, as their romance flourished, talk turned to divorce from their respective spouses. For Carole this was easily achieved; in January 1959 she legally ended her marriage to Jimmy Pappa and resumed her maiden name, Tregoff. Finch, however, had problems.

Although his ardor for Carole was never in doubt, the doctor dragged his heels over divorce action. His tardiness was not inspired by any lingering regard for Barbara—far from it; by this time he detested her—but was, rather, the product of avarice. If Barbara could prove adultery, and there was every indication that she intended to do just that, Finch faced a financial Armageddon. Under California's community property law, Barbara was automatically entitled to half the monies and goods accrued since marriage, but as the aggrieved party in an adultery action she could claim whatever percentage of the community property she saw fit. Californian courts, notorious for siding with the innocent party in such actions, would in all probability accede to her request. This very real likelihood was brought home to Finch in no uncertain manner when Barbara's lawyer filed a claim for 100 percent of her husband's assets, an amount she valued at close to $750,000. In addition she sought $18,000 in legal expenses and alimony of $2,000 a month.

Finch was horrified. He had borrowed heavily to finance his investment in the medical center; if Barbara succeeded in her suit, he would have no alternative but to declare bankruptcy. So he sought to placate his wife, begging her to delay the divorce action for another twelve months, by which time many of his debts with the center would have been settled and he would be on much sounder financial footing.

Barbara told him to go to hell. She was in no mood for conciliation. By this time news of Finch's affair with a girl half his age was common knowledge at the country club. And then there was Carole's malicious insistence on showing up at functions she knew the Finches would be attending together. For Barbara, still slim and attractive but closing in on middle age, such humiliation was unbearable. She could hear the titters at parties, knew she was the butt of a thousand jokes, the subject of endless gossip. Every embarrassment only hardened her intransigence in the divorce settlement. If she couldn't have her husband, then she would damn well have his money!

Finch was at his wits' end. His appeals to Barbara's nonexistent better side became more extreme, more violent. When he heard that she had hired private detectives to secure evidence of his adultery, he telephoned Barbara and suggested a meeting. What began as an adult attempt to discuss mutual grievances went downhill fast. Finch slugged Barbara with a pistol—or so she said later—necessitating a trip to the medical center where he stitched a wound over her eye. (Finch claimed that she had sustained the injury in a fall.) Afterward Barbara went to her lawyer, insisting that he photograph the cut for future reference and also urging him to speed up the divorce proceedings.

On May 18 the couple formally separated. In the days that followed, Barbara went around telling anyone who would listen of Finch's repeated threats to kill her. She was in mortal fear of him, she said, and prayed that he would do nothing to harm her. Three days later she obtained a court order, enjoining Finch to refrain from molesting her, touching family property or withdrawing any funds from the bank beyond those needed for normal business and living expenses. Finch, anticipating the injunction, had withdrawn $3,000 immediately beforehand.

Still anxious not to provide Barbara with evidence of his own infidelity—the divorce papers cited "extreme cruelty" only—Finch moved into a motel. During the next two weeks he visited the house at Lark Hill Drive often, ostensibly to see the children, but also, according to Barbara, to dish out yet more physical abuse to her. This violence took many forms, ranging from assault with miscellaneous implements to one arduous encounter when Finch incapacitated Barbara for several hours by sitting on her chest, a novel but apparently effective means of restraint.

Meanwhile, Barbara continued to broadcast her fears. One friend, a television actor named Mark Stevens, suggested that she get a gun and offered to give her lessons in its use. Barbara did not like the idea but did adopt Stevens's alternative idea of sleeping with a car jack-handle next to her bed. Other friends heard her tell how Finch had threatened to push her off a cliff in a car which would then explode (given the hilly terrain around the matrimonial home, not an unlikely scenario). She spoke of Finch's oft-repeated references to thugs he knew in Las Vegas, men who would kill their own mothers if the price was right.

In the midst of all this animus the couple made one last effort at reconciliation, taking their problems to a marriage counselor. But before any advice was forthcoming from that quarter, Barbara obtained yet another, even more punitive, restraining order in which all Finch's medical-practice income was to be turned over to her for her to dole out as she saw fit. This bombshell sparked off yet another violent confrontation between the warring couple; this only ended when Barbara's Swedish maid, Marie Anne Lindholm, called the police. But before they arrived, Finch had gone. He would be back.

On May 26, perhaps seeking to distance herself from the upheaval to come, Carole moved to Las Vegas. At first she stayed with old family friends until moving into an apartment leased and paid for by Finch. He visited her at every opportunity. To fill up those hours when Finch wasn't around, Carole took a job as a cocktail waitress. Had she restricted herself to this, all might have been well but, through a succession of dubious friends and cronies she gained an introduction to John Patrick Cody, a small-time criminal on the run from a jail sentence in Minneapolis.

Neither could have anticipated just how disastrous that meeting would be.

Glib, oily, entirely bereft of scruple, John Cody had devoted most of his twenty-nine-year existence to a single-minded avoidance of honest endeavor. His police record, depressing in its banality, showed that he had been arrested nineteen times on charges varying from assault and battery to going AWOL from the Marine Corps—and all manner of distractions in between. With his cheap flashy suits, impossibly lubricated hair, white satin ties and padded shoulders, he was a walking caricature of the Hollywood B-movie gangster. Sadly, he lived up to the image. From his conduct both prior and subsequent to meeting Carole Tregoff there is no reason to believe that John Cody had a decent bone in his body.

When he first met Carole it was in his capacity as a self-styled gigolo. She had been scouting all over Vegas for some professional lothario willing to seduce Barbara Finch and thereby provide evidence for a countersuit of adultery. Cody tapped himself on the chest and leeringly assured Carole that her search was over. Just one glance at Cody should have been enough to convince Carole that this was nonsense. Barbara Finch was a sophisticated woman, someone used to the country-club circuit; to picture her falling for a man so obviously flashy and on the make as Jack Cody defied belief. But Cody, slick and unctuous to a quite astonishing degree, managed to convince Carole otherwise. Even more amazingly, he also conned Finch into accepting him as a likely suitor for his estranged wife.

According to Cody, talk of seduction soon turned to plans of an altogether more sinister nature. It was on July 1, he said, that Carole first broached the topic of doing away with Barbara Finch. Cody, who had not the slightest intention of murdering anyone, did however recognize the chance to make a financial killing and immediately quoted a price of $2,000. Carole offered half that amount. After much haggling they settled on $1,400—$350 down, the balance on completion. "I'll need some expenses," said Cody. Carole offered a ticket to Los Angeles. At the same time she provided maps of the house at Lark Hill Drive. The couple discussed what form the murder would take. Cody said that he would arrange it to look as though Mrs. Finch had been killed during a botched robbery.

They agreed upon a date—July 4, Independence Day—so that alibis could be prepared. Carole would be working at the Sands Hotel in Las Vegas. Finch was scheduled to play in a doubles tennis tournament at La Jolla, partnered with a clergyman. Before leaving he told Cody that a shotgun would be stashed in the trunk of his car at Lark Hill Drive.

Cody couldn't believe his good fortune. All his life he'd been looking for a big score; this was it. Pocketing the down-payment, he cashed in the ticket and made a beeline for the nearest casino. After blowing the lot in a crap game, he drove down to Los Angeles for a boozy weekend with one of his many girlfriends. On Sunday, hungover, worn out and broke, he returned to Vegas. Carole was waiting anxiously. How had things gone? she queried. Had he killed Barbara? "Sure," replied Cody, "No problem." Gleefully, Carole handed over an envelope stuffed with one-hundred-dollar bills, then ran to the phone and called Finch with the good news.

Their mutual jubilation lasted twenty-four hours, until a phone call from a very much alive and distressingly healthy Barbara Finch to her astounded husband revealed that something had gone sadly awry.

Another garbled long-distance phone call led to a show-

down between Cody and Carole. Cody professed amazement, insisting that he had, indeed, killed Barbara. Carole
was not impressed. A few hours later Finch arrived hot and
sweating from Los Angeles. One might have expected that
the long desert drive would have further fueled his anger,
yet, incredibly, he gave Cody a very sympathetic hearing.
Cody repeated his story that he had killed some woman
and stuffed her body in the trunk of a car. Finch thought for
a moment and concluded that the victim must have been
one of Barbara's friends. "Jeez," said Cody. "Sorry." After
conning yet another one hundred bucks out of the gullible
doctor, Cody promised to return to Los Angeles and remedy his error.

By this time Cody, realizing that events were spinning
out of control, decided that he had taken these suckers for
every possible penny and promptly headed for Wisconsin,
not to be seen again until Finch and Tregoff were under arrest for murder.

His departure coincided with the blackest of times for
Bernard Finch. For weeks the doctor had been playing cat
and mouse with process servers, always staying just one
step ahead. His luck ran out on July 14 when he was
handed a subpoena alleging contempt of the restraining
order. The order required his attendance in court on July
23, nine days later. Finch crushed the paper to a pulp in his
fist. An awful lot would happen in those nine days.

His life, already hectic, now became an insane swirl, divided between treating patients at the clinic, harassing his
wife at every available opportunity, and plotting her death
in Las Vegas. Whatever resentment Finch felt at being
swindled by Cody was more than outweighed by a burning
determination to fix this problem once and for all. From
this point on Finch acted like a man close to mental col-

lapse. There can be no other reason for the absurdly self-incriminating scheme that he now set into motion.

It began on July 17 when he left his car at Los Angeles airport and caught a flight to Las Vegas. One day later, a Saturday, he and Carole made the return journey to LA in her car. They later claimed that their intent was to confront Barbara with the reality of their relationship—somewhat redundant given the brazenness of their eighteen-month affair—and also to talk her into an out-of-court property-settlement agreement.

Two facts tended to pour cold water on this claim. First was the time of their arrival at Lark Hill Drive—10:00 PM—a suspiciously late hour for such a meeting. Second was the presence in the car of a rather unusual attaché case. Finch later claimed it went everywhere with him and that he found nothing untoward in its contents—a flashlight, two pairs of rubber gloves, some rope, sedatives, two hypodermics with needles, a large carving knife and some .38 caliber ammunition. The police, not without justification, took a rather different view, dubbing the case a "murder kit."

According to the couple, when they arrived at Lark Hill Drive they checked the garage and saw that Barbara's car was missing. To amuse themselves while they waited, and to explain fragments of rubber later found at the crime scene, Carole claimed that she had blown up one of the rubber gloves and played with the Finch's family dog, an elderly Samoyed named Frosty. It was Frosty's rambunctiousness that had caused the glove to tear.

At 11:15 PM Barbara roared up in her red Chrysler. Allegedly Finch went over and began speaking to her. Barbara brought the conversation to a hurried conclusion by drawing a gun. Carole said that Finch then hurled something toward her and told her to run. The something—which turned out to be the infamous attaché case—hit Carole in the stomach and fell to the lawn where it was discovered next day. Carole, heeding Finch's advice, dashed to some bougainvillaea bushes and hid, or so she said. From her sanctuary she could only hear events unfold.

Inside the garage Finch lost all semblance of self-control. All the loathing and hatred he felt toward his wife was distilled into a megadecibel screaming fit. The commotion filtered indoors where the maid, Marie, heard Barbara's cry for help and rushed out to the garage. She saw Finch, poised over his whimpering, semiconscious wife, gun in hand. When Marie became hysterical Finch sought to calm her obvious distress by banging her head repeatedly against the garage wall, hard enough to make a hole in the plaster. Then, to gather everyone's attention—as if such needed to be done—the enraged husband fired one shot at nothing in particular. In the stillness that followed he ordered both women into Barbara's car. Groggily, Marie acquiesced. Barbara was having none of it and hared off down the driveway towards the house next door which belonged to Finch's parents. (Earlier, she had told her lawyer that, in the event of trouble, she would seek shelter at her in-laws.)

While Finch set off in hot pursuit of his fleeing wife, Marie ran back indoors. Just as she grabbed the phone to call the police a second shot rang out.

Sirens wailing, lights ablaze, a horde of patrol cars twisted and swerved their way up the winding road that led to the last house on Lark Hill Drive. As they swung into the driveway the car headlights picked out something unmoving and silent on the ground—the slim body of Barbara Finch.

Never has a murder victim predicted her own demise

with such chilling prescience. Her blonde head, bruised
and bloodied from a brutal pistol-whipping, looked
hideous. But it was the single bullet in the back, exiting between the breasts, that killed her. She was only thirty-six
years old. When the police interviewed Marie, what she
and Barbara's daughter, Patti, had to say pointed in just one
direction. The case seemed iron-clad. All they had to do
was find Dr. Bernard Finch.

Exactly what happened to Finch and Tregoff during the
rest of that night remains one of the most puzzling aspects
of this case. For reasons never fully explained, they became separated. Each made his and her own way back to
Las Vegas, Finch by stolen car. The next day the doctor
was arrested and charged with his wife's murder.
Following a preliminary hearing, Carole Tregoff was similarly charged, and all across America newspaper readers
geared up for what promised to be the juiciest trial in
years.

Whatever bond there was between Carole Tregoff and
Bernard Finch melted in the merciless glare of publicity
that followed their arrest. She spurned his every advance,
returned all the letters he wrote to her in prison unopened
and categorically refused even to acknowledge his existence when their trial began at the packed Los Angeles
County Courthouse on January 4, 1960. Once, when Finch
attempted to kiss her as she brushed past, she neatly side-
stepped, leaving the puckering doctor with a faceful of air
and nothing else. Finch took the slight well. In fact, he
showed very little apprehension at all about his predicament. Prison had taken the edge off his tan, but he still had
that muscular grin, and reporters loved him. To one he expressed surprise that the case should have generated such

interest—journalists had flown in from around the globe to cover the story—then listened intently as she explained why he was such "good copy." "I see," he nodded. "It's partly because I'm an educated man and people wonder. Very interesting . . ." Clearly the doctor's ordeal had done little to undermine his self-confidence.

The first prosecution witness was Marie Anne Lindholm. A shy slender girl caught up in a web of circumstances far beyond her ability to either believe or comprehend, she hesitantly detailed the fateful night's events, then went on to strip away from Finch a good deal of the bonhomie he was struggling to engender. Beneath the smiling veneer, she said, lurked a vicious wife-beater. Over strenuous defense objections, a letter Marie had written before the murder to her mother in Sweden was admitted into evidence. In it she described a thrashing that Finch had given Barbara and his oft-repeated threat that he had hired "someone in Las Vegas" to kill her. Finch could only sit and listen in grim silence. For once his smile failed him. This kind of evidence could put him in the gas chamber.

Defense hopes soared when Jack Cody took the stand. It would take no time at all, they reasoned, to demolish his semiliterate evidence and show him up for the jerk that he was. Except it didn't work out that way. Cody's cheerful admission to just about every form of despicable conduct imaginable—he had been a thief, a sponger, a mugger and occasional swindler—gave his evidence a curious verisimilitude, an honesty that the defense could never quite budge. Attorney Grant Cooper tried hard, but it was useless.

Q.: "What did you do?"
A.: "I loafed."
Q.: "How did you support yourself?"
A.: "By my wit."

Q.: (Later, in reference to one of Cody's girlfriends): "Did she support you?"

A.: "Yes."

Another defense attorney, Rexford Egan, fared no better.

Q.: "Would you lie for money?"

A.: (After a long, thoughtful pause): "It looks like I have."

Cody obviously relished his moment in the limelight. He delivered his answers with a practiced nonchalance, just like all those wiseguys in the movies that he so admired. But there was more to this skinny man than image alone, as he showed when favoring the court with a touching homily, first delivered, so he said, to Finch in an effort to dissuade him from murder: "Killing your wife for money alone isn't worth it . . . let her have every penny . . . take Carole . . . up on a mountaintop and live off the wild. If the girl loves you, she's going to stick with you." Chuckles broke out in the press box. The idea of Jack Cody advocating a solitary existence, sustained only by the fruits of nature, was one which few in court could countenance, let alone swallow.

However, punctuating this sanctimonious claptrap were a few nuggets of pure gold so far as the prosecutors were concerned. By far the most damaging came when Cody detailed a conversation with Carole Tregoff, in which she had snapped: "Jack, you can back out. But if you don't kill her, the doctor will; and if he doesn't, I will!"

By general consensus, when the prosecution rested, prospects looked grim indeed for "The Doctor and the Redhead."

Rumors of a surprise defense counterattack guaranteed a packed courtroom when Finch took the stand. The doctor didn't disappoint. His version of events on the fateful night, coolly delivered, must rank as one of the most original and imaginative fables ever laid before a jury. He began by describing how Barbara had pulled a gun on him. Regrettably, in his efforts to liberate the weapon, he had been forced to club her with it, inflicting two skull fractures. Then, to make matters worse, Marie had entered the garage, screaming her head off. Finch's misconstrued attempts to assuage the maid's obvious distress—already referred to—gave Barbara the chance to snatch up the gun and take off. Finch gave chase. Some way up the drive he saw Barbara taking dead aim at Tregoff with the pistol. A further struggle ensued. Finch grabbed the gun. Barbara began running again. Inexplicably, as Finch attempted to toss the gun away, it went off, neatly drilling his fleeing wife between the shoulder blades. Claiming ignorance of this fact, Finch said he then ran across to his prone wife.

"What happened, Barb?" he cried. "Where are you hurt?"

"Shot . . . in . . . chest," she gasped.

"Don't move a thing . . . I've got to get an ambulance for you and get you to hospital."

Barbara held up a restraining hand. "Wait . . . I'm sorry, I should have listened."

"Barb, don't talk about it now. I've got to get you to hospital."

"Don't leave me. Take care of the kids."

As Finch described feeling for a pulse and finding none, his voice broke. "She was dead." He wiped away a tear. Sobs could also be heard in the public gallery. Others, more hard-boiled, preferred to ponder the likelihood of a murder victim actually apologizing for being shot, and found the story a little thin, to say the least.

Under cross-examination Finch regained his normal

buoyancy. When the prosecutor, referring to numerous affairs with other women before Carole, asked: "Did you tell
these women that you loved them?" the doctor responded
jauntily: "I think under the circumstances that would be
routine."

Seven days on the stand did little to undermine Finch.
He continued to insist that Cody had been nothing more
than a private investigator hired to obtain evidence of
Barbara's infidelity, and that every word of his testimony
was a lie. Finch's story rang hollow, but he stuck to it and
didn't change a word.

This was more than could be said for Carole Tregoff.
Her account changed with the weather. She told an unlikely tale of watching the drama unfold, then cowering for
five or six hours behind some bushes, paralyzed with fear,
while police turned the house upside down. Later, she had
found her car parked on the hill and had driven back to
Vegas alone. Allegedly, her first knowledge of Barbara's
death came via the car radio. When she reached her Vegas
apartment, Finch was already fast asleep in bed. She told
him what she had heard on the radio. He reportedly
shrugged the news off and went back to sleep. Tregoff
went to work.

The prosecution succeeded in making Carole Tregoff
look very bad, intent only on saving herself at the expense
of her former lover. She had, after all, played a leading role
in the solicitation of Cody, and had then given conflicting
stories of why the couple had gone to Lark Hill Drive that
night. Originally, Tregoff told police that the intention was
to talk Barbara out of divorce proceedings. On the stand,
that evolved into an attempt to convince Barbara to obtain
a "quickie" Nevada divorce.

Courtroom observers thought that, at a minimum,
Tregoff's treachery had guaranteed a berth for Finch in San

Quentin's gas chamber. But it was not to be. After eight days of wrangling, the jury declared itself hopelessly deadlocked and a mistrial was declared. Apparently, all the jurors believed the existence of a Las Vegas conspiracy to kill Barbara Finch, but some refused to convict Finch and Tregoff because Cody was not charged also. It later transpired that racial tension—one jury member was black, another Hispanic—had led to ugly scenes in the jury room when neither minority juror would yield to pressure exerted by their white counterparts.

Any mistrial always favors the accused. Memories fade, occasionally witnesses die and doubts are often planted in the minds of subsequent jurors. This was borne out at the second trial which also ended in deadlock, despite an extraordinary admonition to the jury by Judge LeRoy Dawson who thundered, in no uncertain terms, that they ought not to believe a single word uttered by either defendant.

With the case of Finch and Tregoff rapidly assuming the status of a second-rate soap opera, prosecutors despaired of ever finding twelve citizens willing to convict this couple of murder. Finally they decided to change tack. In the third trial, more restrained than its predecessors, the evidence concentrated less on sex and moral judgements, more on facts. Stripped of its sensationalism the case was every bit as straightforward as prosecutors had initially thought, with the result that, on March 27, 1961, Dr. Bernard Finch was convicted of murder in the first degree; Carole Tregoff in the second. Both received life imprisonment.*

---

*In 1969 Carole Tregoff was paroled from prison. She changed her name and found work at a hospital in the Pasadena area. Finch, released two years later, spent a decade practicing medicine in Missouri before returning to Covina in 1984.

• • •

The sentences caused outrage as citizens wondered how such premeditated killers could have escaped the gas chamber. At that time California was a bastion of capital punishment; after all, just ten months earlier, convicted kidnapper Caryl Chessman (following twelve well-publicized years on death row) had been executed, more for humiliating the legal system than for anything else. And neither was California one of those states that have traditionally shown leniency to women. So why did Finch and Tregoff escape the ultimate penalty? True, three trials helped dilute public opprobrium and the memory of what they had done, but there was more at work here than mere delay. It had to do with the defendants themselves. Historically, the record shows that, if one is on trial for one's life in an American courtroom, a handsome appearance is no bad thing to have. A well-respected occupation doesn't hurt, either.

11. A NEW YEAR'S RESOLUTION

The woman showed no signs of stirring. Ever since the operation she had lain unconscious in her hospital bed in Bromley, just south of London, pumped full of sedatives, barely breathing, barely alive. Throughout the ordeal her husband had been a model of concern and solicitousness, always on hand bearing gifts. Today it was a bouquet of flowers. As he paced the small private room, his fleshy sensuous face creased in a frown. Being a doctor he was no stranger to hospitals, but never under these circumstances. His hands worked nervously together, almost as if praying. He kept darting quick glances at the comatose woman. At other times his eyes caught the gaze of the police officer who had stayed at the woman's side ever since her operation. There was sympathy in the officer's face, but there was something else, a determination to preserve his professional detachment. It was his job to be there when the woman woke. The hospital doctors had warned him not to expect too much. Besides the physical atrocities she had undergone, there was the mental trauma as well. Would she even remember who her attackers were?

On the third day the woman's eyes flickered. After a monumental effort, they blinked open. She stared round at the strange room, trying to focus. Sluggishly she took in her surroundings. Then she saw her husband. As his round smiling face bent toward her, she shrank back into her pillow. Her mouth opened to speak but nothing came out. As the doctors feared, the attack had left her literally speechless.

Under the officer's watchful gaze, the husband leaned down and whispered a few words into his wife's ear. The officer was no linguist but he guessed that the strange-sounding language was Hindi, the couple's native tongue. He couldn't help but notice, though, the strange expression that drained the woman's face of all color. The husband kept talking, low, urgent. All the time the smile remained fixed—or was it forced?—on his face. The officer wasn't sure. Not wanting to intrude, he remained silent, absorbing, attentive. After some minutes he saw the woman move her head ever so slightly, as if nodding in agreement. The effect on her husband was palpable. A gleam lightened the previously anxious eyes as he stood back from the bed, something approaching triumph on his face.

Shortly afterward, saying that his wife should rest, he left the room, his step sprightly and sure. No sooner had he gone than the woman frantically motioned the officer toward her. She began to gesticulate wildly, a grotesque pantomime. From her movements the officer realized that she wanted a pencil and paper. He found both. In a barely legible hand the woman scratched out a short message, handed it to the officer, then fell back into an exhausted sleep.

Just a dozen words, but with them forty-three-year-old

Madhu Baksh purged herself of a dreadful secret about the man she had married. Looking down, the officer flinched: "My husband John is a killer. He killed his first wife, too."

Good God! How, he wondered, could it have come to this?

The events leading up to that hospital-room encounter had their genesis several years earlier in 1979. At that time John Baksh, the Indian-born son of a clergyman, was still married to his first wife, Ruby. Both were doctors and very successful. They shared joint partnerships in two South London practices, one in Mottingham, an area of broad social mix, and another in the more affluent suburb of Chislehurst. The husband-and-wife doctor team were respected members of the community, prosperous and happy. Patients and friends knew John Baksh as a kind and gentle man, a perfect husband and father to the couple's two adopted children. He had a sleek, well-fed air of affluence about him, a man who had made plenty of money and wasn't shy about flaunting it. Ruby was less outgoing but equally ambitious. Asked for an opinion, most would have described the Bakshs as an ideal couple.

And so they were until another young doctor joined the practice in 1979. Madhu Kumar was shy and petite and struggling to free herself from a desperate plight. Ten years earlier she had arrived in England from her native Lucknow, straight into the misery of an arranged marriage. The prompt arrival of two children, a boy and a girl, did nothing to aid this loveless union. Madhu suffered in miserable silence. For a doctor of such spectacular qualifications—she was a fellow of the Royal College of Surgeons of Edinburgh and a member of the Royal College of Gynaecologists—the situation was doubly dreadful. At work she was a champion, at home little more than a chattel, penalized by ancient custom and tradition. Freedom came just after joining the Baksh practice when she was finally granted a separation from her husband. After that, all she wanted was to get on with her life, her career and her children.

But someone else already had designs on this attractive young woman.

Dr. John Baksh had never made any great effort to conceal the lust he felt towards his junior partner. Each time Madhu turned around he was there, lingering and looking, always looking. In this fashion the doctor began a slow, measured seduction, one that would take years. Flattery and compliments led to more suggestive comments, then to blunt propositions. Madhu had no trouble deflecting all of this. The rejections didn't seem to bother Baksh, each one only emboldened his approach. One night he arrived unannounced at Madhu's flat in Bromley, brandishing a bottle of bubbly. He also came armed with some stinging sarcasm about Madhu's strict Hindu upbringing, pointing out that she was in England now and should adopt a more permissive attitude. All the while he plied her with champagne. It served him poorly. Madhu's generosity extended to preparing dinner and nothing more. Then she showed Baksh the door.

Daunted but not defeated, the doctor assured himself that it was only a matter of time before Madhu unlocked her heart. He just needed to find the right key. He tried flowers, jewelry, clothes. None of it worked. Madhu cold-shouldered every advance. Baksh fumed and redoubled his efforts.

"He never gave up," said Madhu later. "He tried to kiss and caress me. He told me how much he loved me and how he would die if I persisted in refusing. Then he would break down weeping. He was good at that . . ."

As Baksh's obsession festered, discretion flew out of the window. He abandoned all hopes of keeping Ruby in the dark; nothing else mattered except his determination to bed Madhu.

For Ruby Baksh it was a dagger in the heart, watching her husband's blinkered pursuit of this younger woman. Anger gave way to tears, tears gave way to humiliation, until a black cloak of depression wrapped itself around her. Apart from the emotional devastation there were other factors. The family finances were in desperate shape, the result of Baksh squandering thousands on his obsession. By November 1982 Ruby's despair had driven her to the brink of suicide.* She was convinced her husband was sleeping with Madhu. Baksh would have been only too delighted if this were the case but, apart from what he termed "kissing and cuddling sessions," he had still not made any significant progress with Madhu. She flatly refused to entertain any suggestion of an affair while he was still married to Ruby. Get a divorce, said Madhu, and we'll take it from there.

Just four weeks after this ultimatum Baksh took Ruby and their two children on holiday to their villa in Turre in southern Spain. They planned to stay over Christmas and the New Year. Ruby saw this as a chance—maybe her last—to win back the man she loved. She was determined not to miss it.

It turned out to be the most miserable Christmas of her life. The couple argued constantly. Baksh, while hotly denying Ruby's allegations of infidelity, made it plain that he was no longer interested in keeping their marriage alive.

*Baksh later claimed that Ruby had actually taken a drug overdose but had been caught in time.

Ruby wept helplessly, more convinced than ever that her husband was a brazen adulterer.

As the last days of 1982 crept painfully by, Ruby Baksh felt ever more bereft. She had little stomach for the New Year's Eve party planned at a local bar; nevertheless, she resolved to go. Wearing her bravest face, she entered the festivities on the arm of her husband. The bar was packed. Among the other guests was Paul Polanski, brother of noted movie director, Roman Polanski. He remembered later that Ruby had seemed to be in good spirits, as had Baksh. In fact the couple couldn't have appeared happier. After midnight, when the party broke up, they returned laughing and joking to their villa. Next morning the holiday enclave received stunning news—Dr. Ruby Baksh, aged thirty-six, was dead.

With neither Baksh nor the local police speaking the other's language, Polanski was called in to act as interpreter. In an extravagantly lachrymose performance, Baksh claimed that Ruby's heart, already feeble, had not been up to the strenuous party. She had collapsed suddenly, he sobbed. When the police said that they required confirmation of this diagnosis from a local doctor, Baksh suggested an elderly man he had met socially. The doctor was summoned and, through Polanski, spoke with Baksh. Polanski said, "The Spanish doctor asked how his wife was the night before—if she had had any illness. He [Baksh] said his wife had said something about not feeling too well." In the absence of any contradictory symptoms and under Baksh's gentle but firm coaxing, the local doctor duly signed a death certificate, citing heart failure.

Baksh's next move was peculiar. Over the vehement opposition of her family, he insisted on Ruby being buried in Spain. He gave no reason for this, other than convenience.

Upon receipt of the undertaker's bill, though, Baksh flew into a rage over what he considered outlandishly high funeral expenses, but he paid them anyway. More than anything he seemed anxious to throw a blanket over the whole affair. He had good cause.

Just days after her death, a letter written by Ruby Baksh arrived in India at the home of her sister, Janet Williams, a nurse. In it Ruby said, "I am fed up and I am going to commit suicide." Desperate to avoid the public shame of a suicide in the family, Mrs. Williams immediately destroyed the letter.

In the light of this letter much of Baksh's unseemly haste in expediting the funeral arrangements, and particularly the death certificate, takes on fresh significance. Unbeknownst to Mrs. Williams, or anyone else except her husband, Ruby Baksh was worth a great deal of money dead, providing that death had been natural and unprovoked. She had life insurance coverage of £90,000, with her husband as the sole beneficiary. Since the merest hint of suicide would have attracted a whole swarm of suspicious claims adjusters, Baksh, in serious financial difficulties, had to conceal the actual cause of death or risk not receiving a penny. Unaware of the insurance policy, Mrs. Williams believed that Baksh was acting from a similar motive as herself, a desire to avoid the stigma of suicide. For this reason she vowed to keep the news to herself.

Someone else, however, already had suspicions that all was not as it seemed with the death of Ruby Baksh.

By pure chance another Bromley resident had been in Turre over the New Year. Restaurant owner Barry Willmott knew Baksh only fleetingly but was struck by how indifferent the doctor seemed to the tragedy. Hardly the reaction of a bereaved husband, thought Willmott. Just as quickly the idea slipped away, relegated to the back of his mind where it would remain dormant for years, only to be awakened in the strangest and most horrific fashion.

Baksh, meanwhile, returned with the children to England. Madhu was waiting for him at Gatwick Airport. As he came through customs and immigration and into the arrivals lounge, Baksh wore a black hat and was weeping profusely. Madhu's heart went out to him in his time of bereavement. She agreed to look after him and his two children until he had recovered from the shock. Baksh blubbered his gratitude, barely able to restrain his elation. The long wait was nearly over.

Two weeks later Baksh moved one step nearer his goal. In a bizarre ceremony at Madhu's flat he first swore his undying love. Then, with the sickly sweet scent of incense hanging heavy in the air, Madhu knelt in submission at Baksh's feet as he placed his dead wife's wedding ring on her finger and the couple exchanged vows.

One week later the union was consummated.

It proved to be everything the doctor had hoped for.

Dr. John Baksh returned to his twin practices. He was on top of the world. He had a new mistress, £90,000 in his pocket, and an unholy ambition to elevate himself up the social ladder. More than anything else Baksh yearned for entrée into the circles of privilege and wealth. An unmitigated snob, he took the proceeds from Ruby's insurance policy and went house hunting. Not just any house, that wasn't his style; it had to be something special. He found it in the decorous suburb of Bickley, deep in stockbroker territory. The house, an imposing brick-built monument to the good life, stood its ground in one of Bickley's most exclusive roads, and was worth a cool £250,000 even before the eighties house price explosion. Intensely ambitious and determined to impress the hell out of any visitor, Baksh went on a decorating binge, lavishing thousands on deep-pile luxury carpets and the finest furniture he could find. The man who had balked at paying his wife's funeral bill didn't hesitate to plunge £15,000 into redecorating just two bathrooms. The taps were gold-plated, the semicircular tub was pure Sunday supplement, no expense spared, first class all the way.

It was the same in his social life; Baksh did nothing by halves. In May 1983 he and Madhu journeyed to Paris for a brief holiday. They booked into a Montparnasse hotel. The trip was something of a recovery mission: already the first cracks were beginning to appear in their relationship. Fights had broken out almost daily as Baksh's desire to please Madhu became borderline psychotic. This made his sudden coolness on the trip so difficult for Madhu to fathom. It worsened through the holiday. He seemed distant, as though plagued by worry. Verification came one morning when, after she had got up, he called her back to bed. His eyes filled with those familiar tears that he seemed able to conjure up at will. She asked him what was the matter. Baksh peered long into her face. At last he spoke. In a hesitant, often tremulous voice, Dr. John Baksh dropped his bombshell—Ruby had not committed suicide at all . . . he had killed her.

Madhu shrank away. Her heart thumped against the wall of her ribcage. Oh God, no. This couldn't be happening! She stared at the man who sat propped up in bed. He seemed much calmer now, talking as if nothing had happened; how each night he would take Ruby a cup of hot milk, but on that New Year's Eve he had spiked her drink with a sleeping potion. Once she was unconscious a massive injection of morphine into her thigh had finished her off. It was a quiet death, he insisted; she had not suffered at all. Baksh concluded by saying, "What I have done is the biggest sacrifice anyone can make for love."

Madhu begged him to explain.

He whined, "If I had not done so, I would not have got you!"

Then it was time for the tears again. Not so intense as before, and certainly not enough to prevent him from turning over and falling into a deep sleep.

As Madhu sat on the side of the bed, a million thoughts raced through her mind. Fury, disbelief, depression but, most of all, fury. Her first marriage had been a disaster; now she had been duped into giving herself to a murderer.

The more she thought about it the more incensed she became. She wanted to run outside and scream out loud on the streets of Paris that John Baksh was a brutal killer. She wanted him locked away forever. But who would believe her? He was a highly respected doctor. Doctors didn't murder people! It would be just her word against his. Slowly, almost imperceptibly, the fury gave way to an insidious fear. If he had killed once, what was to stop him killing again? A chill ran through her body as she gazed down at the snoring figure beside her. She was trapped. All she could do was keep this dreadful secret locked away in a dark, untenanted corner of her memory and pray that it would never again see the light of day.

When Baksh awoke it was as though nothing had happened. Madhu tried hard to convince herself that it had all been a bad dream. She almost succeeded. Not quite, but enough so that, when her own divorce was finalized, Madhu officially became the second Mrs. Baksh. The wedding was held on January 7, 1984. The groom smiled a lot at the ceremony. January was getting to be his lucky month.

•   •   •

When, much later, she was challenged for having know-
ingly married a murderer, Madhu Baksh offered no excuses, just an illumination of her own thought processes. "I
did not think of him as a murderer after a time. I think he
was a human being who had made a big mistake, for which
he was ashamed . . . He said God had forgiven him."

It was this attitude that she took into the marriage and
the practice, to which she became an increasingly valuable
addition. The couple prospered. Between them, husband
and wife grossed an annual income in excess of £80,000,
handsome by most standards, peanuts for someone of John
Baksh's extravagance. Always a smooth dresser himself,
he set about remaking Madhu in the image of what he
thought the British upper-crust housewife should look like.
On one shopping expedition to Harrods, Baksh told Madhu
to pick out any dress she wanted. Once she had decided, he
ordered the assistant to bring four more, just like it. Baksh
set enormous store by material possessions, convinced that
gifts were the answer to every problem. Whenever he and
Madhu argued, which was often, he would attempt to make
up by buying her another present. But he was caught in a
vicious circle. The more he sought to buy off Madhu, the
more his free-spending ways left a trail of unpaid bills,
adding to the acrimony in the marriage.

By the end of 1985 Dr. John Baksh was fifty-three years
old, holding his marriage together with masking tape, and
up to his eyes in debt. He owed the Inland Revenue £6,000
in back taxes, the bank was hounding him to reduce a bal-
looning overdraft, and his children were in very real danger of having to leave the private school they attended
because their father could not meet the fees. Despite all
this, not once would Baksh acknowledge his financial in-
sufficiencies, or the deleterious effect they had on his mar-

riage. He had, in common with countless other murderers, infinite powers of rationalization. It was always Madhu's fault. Speaking later, Baksh said they "got on well generally, but things were very bad at times. This was caused by her bad temper. We had fights, it almost came to blows."

Ominously, no matter how serious his financial woes, there was one item that Baksh always managed to find money for—insurance premiums. Although she didn't know it, Madhu was a walking gold mine like the first Mrs. Baksh. Baksh kept increasing the cover on her life until, by December 1985, he had taken out policies totaling £215,000. The premiums were eating him alive, £1,000 per month, or one sixth of the family income, but Baksh somehow coped. Besides, the policies were an investment—one that could pay off at any time.

Each passing month pushed their marriage that much nearer to the brink of disaster. The rows, always mean, now took on a newfound frequency and viciousness. Things came to a head in the first week of January 1986 when, during one brutal exchange, Madhu yelled at Baksh that she was going to the police with the truth about Ruby's death. Baksh froze. He had not heard this before. The threat silenced him. Throughout the remainder of that week he brooded. But on Saturday, January 4, the row erupted again. All day long the couple drank champagne and spit venom at each other. In between rows they managed an outing in the car. The day was icy cold and neither wanted to stay out long. It was just after they had pulled into the driveway of their house that Baksh noticed a mark on Madhu's eyelid. He leant across for a closer look.

After that Madhu remembered nothing.

•　　•　　•

Keith Corbett was going to see for himself. The forty-six-year-old naturalist had heard the stories—wholesale butchery down at Keston Ponds—and it made his blood boil. This skein of tiny lakes tucked away in the Kent countryside, some twenty miles south of London, had always been a popular late-night rendezvous for courting couples in cars, but just lately careless drivers had been running down toads by the dozen, even the occasional badger. It definitely needed looking into.

Corbett was a man who took his ecology seriously. How else could his presence at Keston Ponds be explained on what would be the coldest night of the year? It was the moon that had brought him out, full and brilliant, perfect for his needs. Undaunted by the subzero temperatures, he crept stealthily along the narrow lane that bisected the ponds. On either side of the road dense undergrowth stretched far into the night, too thick even for the brilliant shafts of moonlight to penetrate. Off to his left eddies of mist swirled across the still water. The silence was unearthly. Corbett tuned his ear for the toad's distinctive croak. Experience told him that he was likeliest to find them on a brush-covered hillock known locally as Caesar's Bank.

He picked his path cautiously, avoiding an area of frosty grass that would crunch underfoot, and worked his way along the bank toward a cluster of holly bushes. Suddenly he stopped in his tracks, hairs prickling the nape of his neck. As he later described it: "I heard a wheezing noise. At first I thought it was an injured fox. Then I went closer . . ."

Slowly his eyes adjusted to the murk. He gently eased a cluster of prickly holly leaves to one side. The sound was louder now, an odd hissing, like something gasping for breath. He finally located the source, an indistinct shape lying on the ground. Not some wounded animal, he was sure of that. He looked more closely. At last the picture came into focus. It was a woman, small, dark-haired, motionless. "I saw her legs sticking out. My initial reaction was that she was a drunk."

Corbett shone his flashlight on the comatose woman, then recoiled as if struck by a jolt of electricity. "There was blood everywhere. It was a horrific sight."

Indeed it was. Someone had opened up the woman's throat with a knife.

Earlier that evening, around nine-thirty, the police station in nearby Bromley had received a phone call from John Baksh. The doctor was in a state of high agitation. He explained that Madhu had left their house at 5:00 PM to do some shopping but had not returned home. Concerned, Baksh and his brother-in-law, Dhruva Kumar, had gone looking for her, but found only her silver Ford Orion abandoned in Bromley's town center near the magistrate's court. Baksh squealed that she must have been the victim of abductors, only something so ghastly could have prevented his beloved from returning home on tonight of all nights when they planned to celebrate their second wedding anniversary!

Quite understandably the police did not evince any great concern. Such calls are a daily occurrence. Most are the product of domestic disputes, beyond their province unless actual harm befalls one of the parties. Even the fact that Baksh was a doctor did not generate alarm; after all, even physicians are not immune to the odd matrimonial bust-up. The police soothed Baksh, told him that his call had been logged, but regretted that there was nothing they could do until at least forty-eight hours had elapsed.

•   •   •

Thrusting his way through the bushes, Keith Corbett blundered out to the lane. He began running. Faster. There were houses nearby, no more than a half mile away. He could find help there. His breath billowed on the frigid night air. His lungs felt as if they were about to burst. He reached the houses. Most stood in darkness. He finally found one with its lights on. Behind the windows a belated New Year's Eve dinner party was underway, all brightness and laughter. Corbett raced up and pounded on the door.

With fast-diminishing disbelief the hostess listened as this wild-eyed intruder panted out his fantastic story. While one of the guests dialed 999, the others, clad in their party finery, followed Corbett back to Caesar's Bank.

The frozen woman was still alive but only just. They wrapped her in a blanket, as much to block out the horror of that gaping windpipe as to keep her warm, then took turns to rub some life into the victim's icy hands, all the while assuring her that help was on its way.

Within minutes an ambulance arrived. The emergency crew did what they could then rushed the stricken woman to hospital. All through the night surgeons worked to seal the hideous five-inch gash. Whatever caused this terrible wound had severed muscles, nerves, tendons, blood vessels and chipped the jawbone. After several hours of the most painstaking and intricate surgery, the woman was finally stabilized. One doctor estimated that she would have been dead in another thirty minutes. That she had already survived so long was a miracle, attributable, of all things, to that night's intense cold. Hypothermia had slowed the body's metabolism almost to a standstill and, with it, the blood loss. A few degrees warmer and she would have been long gone. There were other factors as well but they wouldn't become apparent until later.

No great feats of detection were required to establish that the victim was the missing Dr. Madhu Baksh. Yet when police informed her husband his reaction seemed curiously ambivalent. The overwhelming relief that police had been expecting was not there. In its place . . . well, it was difficult to say, but it was certainly odd.

While Madhu lay unconscious in hospital next day, recovering from the emergency operation, Baksh persisted in his story of kidnappers. As a theory it sounded plausible. Baksh dressed expensively and well. So did Madhu. They moved in wealthy circles. An interested party might well conclude from observing this doctor couple pull up to their front door in a gleaming new BMW that here was an ideal opportunity for kidnap and ransom. Certainly the police took Baksh's story seriously enough to appeal through the press for any witnesses to the abduction to contact them. None did. All the police could do was wait for Madhu Baksh to regain consciousness.

When the sedation finally wore off and she opened her eyes, Madhu's first vision was of her husband. As she later put it: "He had a bouquet of flowers and was leaning down giving me a look of love . . . he asked me if I could remember the masked men around my car." Whispering in Hindi, Baksh kept reminding her that she had been abducted from outside the Army and Navy stores in Bromley. She went on,

> I was unable to speak but I shook my head as if to say no. I lifted my finger to show there was one man. I pointed at him. He started to plead. He said, "Save me, save my life, otherwise I will go to jail." I wanted to push him away but my mind said no. He must not think I would not cooperate, and I was worried about the children.

Once she had convinced Baksh that she would accede to his demands, she watched him go, then begged the police officer for a piece of paper and a pencil.

All through her convalescence Madhu remained under a twenty-four-hour police guard. During this period Baksh acted like a madman. He embarked on an extraordinary letter-writing campaign aimed at getting Madhu to change her story; the content of these letters leaves considerable doubt about the writer's state of mind. In one he begged, "My darling Madhu. I am very sorry for what happened— that I put a knife to your throat. I did not know what I was doing and hope that you soon recover. Children are fine, love ever, John."

When this failed to elicit any favorable sort of reaction he tried again. "We are both alive. It is a storm in a teacup. Worse could have happened. I need psychiatric help." Mercifully Baksh spared Madhu details of just how much "worse" it could have been.

Baksh's arrest for attempted murder sent shockwaves through the uneventful and reserved community where he lived. Customers at a local restaurant could talk of little else. Eventually the proprietor, his interest piqued, picked up a copy of the local newspaper. Barry Willmott studied the accused man's photograph and cast his mind back three years to Turre in Spain. It was the same face all right, no doubt about that. Perhaps he ought to inform the police?

Together with Madhu's own incredible story, Willmott's intervention convinced the authorities to open an inquiry into the circumstances of Ruby Baksh's death. Pathologists from the Home Office were despatched to Spain with orders to exhume the dead woman's body.

When Baksh heard this news he grabbed his pen and

dashed off yet another of his manic epistles to Madhu. "The whole world is against us and our love. I wish I had wings to fly to you and put things right. What I told you about Ruby was not right. I only muttered things about her to make you love me even more."

When the pathologists arrived in Spain they received some unexpectedly good news. Before interment in the coffin, Ruby Baksh's body had been wrapped in plastic sheeting. This kept it in a far better state of preservation than could otherwise have been expected. Samples from the liver and other organs extracted for examination were found to contain fatal amounts of morphine.

This did not, of course, contradict Baksh's story that Ruby had committed suicide after learning that he and Madhu were having an affair. He explained to the police: "I told her [Ruby] I would try and break off the relationship but Ruby was upset and very hurt. After returning from a New Year's party she was sad and pensive."

Baksh said that he found a note beside his wife's body which declared, "I cannot take it anymore. I am afraid I have to go. This time I am making sure I will not wake up."

"So what about the confession in Paris?" asked detectives. Baksh gave a nervous giggle. That had all been a concoction on his part, designed to impress his new lover. "It was very foolish of me. I suppose I was trying to get favor from her. I was trying to convey to her that I loved her very much and would do anything for her. Of course it was not true—I did not do it . . . I told her that I had given Ruby a morphine injection." Baksh insisted that two weeks later he recanted the story to Madhu, saying it had all been a fabrication; he had not killed Ruby at all.

Then how did Madhu come to be lying under a holly bush with her throat slashed open?

Baksh had an answer for that one as well. Again, it had

all been Madhu's fault, he said, the result of a daylong champagne-and-shouting marathon. At one point, according to Baksh, she had "rushed to the kitchen and come back with a knife. She said she was going to cut my throat. I grabbed it out of her hand and tried to calm her down."

All this alcohol and unremitting conflict clearly had an unsettling effect on Madhu. When she complained of an intense pain in her chest Baksh said he gave her a morphine injection with her consent. Suitably revived, Madhu renewed hostilities. Baksh, in desperation, suggested that they seek advice on their relationship from some police friends who lived in nearby Biggin Hill. Baksh said that he took the knife with him so he could show the friends "just how serious things had got."

"When we got to Keston Ponds I wanted to stop. I thought if we both got some fresh air we would be better. I helped her over a fence and wanted her to sit down. Suddenly she said, 'Where's the knife?' I thought she was just hallucinating. I made her sit down near a bush, then I foolishly went back to the car and brought the knife. In my mind I thought: I would demonstrate to her what it was like—how it felt—to have someone point a knife at someone's throat and threaten them. I told her, 'There's your knife.' She pushed it with her left hand. It all happened in a split second."

Inadvertently the knife ripped a gash five inches wide across Madhu's throat. Baksh insisted that he had just pointed the knife at her neck "to teach her a lesson or whatever." He concluded this nonsense with the extraordinary remark that he had not considered Madhu's injury to be that serious, and thought that she might walk home unaided!

· · ·

Needless to say, the police version of that day's events ran along rather different lines. They hypothesized that, when Baksh and Madhu arrived home, he had secretly injected his wife with some form of drug. Madhu had no recollection of being carried indoors where Baksh once again injected her, this time with a near-lethal dose of morphine in the thigh. He waited until dark, then carried her back to the car and bundled her into the trunk. Pausing only to grab a foot-long knife from the kitchen, Baksh drove off into the night.

He reached Keston Ponds in the early evening. He had chosen his time well. This renowned lovers' lane would not attract its usual quota of the impassioned and the inflamed until much later on. For now he was safe. Lugging Madhu's body up onto Caesar's Bank, he stuffed it beneath a holly bush, then set to with his carefully scripted plan for murder.

If doctors are supposed to be able to kill cleverly, then Baksh did not disappoint. This was close to being a perfect murder. He knew that the subzero January temperature and the morphine would combine to slow Madhu's metabolism to a fraction of its normal rate. All he had to do was take the kitchen knife, saw across her jugular vein in such a way that she would bleed slowly, and he could be miles away creating an alibi when she actually expired. This is exactly what he did. But Baksh was too clever. That night the temperature plunged precipitously, much farther than he had anticipated. Madhu's functions slowed almost to a standstill. But it was a close-run business. That his plan did not succeed was due entirely to one man's concern for toads and badgers.

At his trial at the Central Criminal Court in London, Baksh faced charges of murdering Ruby and attempting to murder

Madhu. The prosecution speculated that, having success-fully disposed of one wife for a huge cash settlement, Baksh was confident of repeating the feat. The attempt on Madhu's life, they maintained, was motivated by greed alone. Totaling up the insurance policies and balancing them against Baksh's known financial difficulties left a handsome residue, one that could have lasted years, even for this free spender. (Ironically, one policy, worth £60,000, was taken out so recently that the actual policy document did not arrive until after Madhu was in the hospital.)

The main prosecution witness was Baksh's intended second victim. Wearing a high-necked dress to cover her scarred throat, and without once looking at her husband in the dock, Madhu Baksh could only tell her story in a whis-per. The attack had severed her vocal chords and left her tongue partially paralyzed but she had breath enough to slam the cell door on her husband.*

Baksh's own performance was dismal. Any inventive-ness he showed in the manner of his crime entirely de-serted him under the prosecution's withering assault. He lied, prevaricated, then lied again, often in the same sen-tence. Even his own counsel had difficulty swallowing some of the drivel that Baksh spouted, especially his ad-mission that, when he had returned to the bank to pick up a bloodstained glove, Madhu was still lying in the same position on the grass, breathing normally. "Why, in heaven's name, didn't you telephone for an ambulance or take her to a hospital?" asked Queen's Counsel Robin Simpson incredulously.

---

*The authorities declined to charge Madhu Baksh with being an acces-sory to murder because they considered that she had suffered enough. They also doubted their ability to prove that she believed her husband's confession.

All Baksh could do was mumble, "I couldn't think properly." He said that he couldn't face a scandal about two respectable doctors drinking to excess, taking drugs and quarreling. He did not want anyone to know their "dark secrets."

On December 18, 1986, the doctor was convicted on both counts. He stood, hands clasped together in prayer and close to tears, as the recorder of London, Sir James Miskin, sentenced him to life imprisonment with a recommendation that he serve at least twenty years for killing Ruby. He was also given a concurrent jail term of fourteen years for the attempted murder of Madhu.

Dr. John Baksh knew full well the evil that breathed inside him. Before standing trial he had confirmed his Jekyll and Hyde personality to police officers: "It was the animal in me that wanted to kill her." Even so, any remorse he showed arose more from his own predicament than regret at what he had done. About the best he could offer by way of apology came when he said, almost as an afterthought, "One doesn't realize the importance of a person until their absence." Strange words, indeed, for a would-be double murderer.

12. THREE MEN IN A HURRY

The last time any disinterested party saw Ellis Henry Greene alive, the thirty-two-year-old Los Angeles bookkeeper was drunker than hell. For most patrons jammed inside the Bullet, a heaving gay bar on Hollywood's Burbank Boulevard, his condition hardly warranted a second glance. Greene was someone who liked his drink, even if it didn't much like him, and most nights he could be relied on to get drunk. Tonight, though, he was especially legless. He had plenty to celebrate: tax deadline day—April 15— always a pain for anyone in the accountancy business, had passed without a hitch. Now it was time to relax and sink a few.

As the evening wore on, Greene's manic drinking stoked up the other great preoccupation of his life—sex. He bounced around the club like a pinball, flirting desperately with anyone who would pay attention and with some who wouldn't. If his barroom conduct was outrageous then his appearance was not: medium build, medium height, medium-brown hair. Just about everything about Ellis

Greene was medium, except his capacity for booze and sex.

The drinking was a recent habit. Back home in Ohio, family members knew Ellis as just one of seven kids at the dinner table, easy to overlook, a quiet, undemonstrative boy who grew into a quiet, undemonstrative man. His marriage survived several uneventful years and then abruptly collapsed when, to general astonishment, Greene announced that he was gay. With the admission came a new lease on life and a desire to be free from midwestern parochialism.

In 1985 he moved to California into the North Hollywood home of his aunt. By day he worked for a San Fernando Valley accountant; at night he cruised the bars. His breakneck promiscuity, in a milieu where casual sex was commonplace and rarely commented on, became notorious. Ellis Greene liked his sex rough and he liked it often, several men a night. To some he sold hard-core porn as a means of supplementing his income; others bought his company with drinks in anticipation of the sadomasochistic extravaganza to come. The lifestyle did have its compensations. In early April Greene had excitedly phoned his brother in Ohio with the news that he had just met two entrepreneurs who were interested in investing in a long-cherished dream of his, a cheesecake company that would market his own special recipe. It promised to be a real moneymaker. They seemed genuinely excited.

But there was no sign of either investor on this particular Friday night in 1988. Greene's bleary eyes scanned the crowd. Maybe they were at some other bar? He drank up. It was 11:30 PM. As Ellis Greene, always drunk, always horny, lurched unsteadily out into the cool California night, other customers waved or shouted their good-byes. Some smiled, some shook their heads, little realizing that they would never see Ellis Greene alive again. No one would, except the person who murdered him.

Eighteen months earlier, in late 1986, three men had begun putting the final touches to a complex plan designed to ensure their complete financial independence. They rarely met—most of the scheming was done by phone—but any casual observer who saw them together might have thought them an ill-matched trio. Two were in business together, yet it was they who seemed the most dissimilar. The older man, Melvin Hanson, was rangy and thin, with an artfully arranged fringe of grayish-yellow hair that tried (but never quite succeeded) in covering the balding pate beneath. His haggard face and hacking cough, brought on by a three-pack-a-day cigarette habit, made him seem years older than his actual age of forty-four. Despite his unprepossessing appearance nearly everyone who met him commented on his soft-spoken charm. It had served him handsomely in his well-paid job as a buyer for a chain of shoestores. Most would have been happy with the annual salary of $75,000. But not Hanson. He was hungry for more. In 1981, he found it.

That was the year he met John Barrett Hawkins, a brash and brawny six footer, still only nineteen, with shoulder-length curly dark hair and icy blue eyes, the kind of Greek-god looks that drew gasps from women and men alike. This suited the young man's ambivalent sexuality well. Hawkins had honed his hustling skills working as a bartender at Studio 54 in New York City; there he let it be known that his rock-hard body, sculpted by long hours in the gym, was available for a price. At $5,000 a night, if the client could afford it, Hawkins's price was also negotiable, $50 sometimes, confirming the belief that it was hustling Hawkins was addicted to, not money. Besides, he made a lot of money dealing drugs, quaaludes mostly, which he bought at two dollars a tab from a doctor in Los Angeles, then resold to the club's well-heeled clientele for ten times that figure.

Sexual attraction drew Hanson to Hawkins; mutual greed kept them together. Each fancied himself an entrepreneur but, first, they needed some seed money. That came when Hawkins rented a ton of expensive furniture for his apartment, then called a removals company and told them to come and pick everything up. Once the furniture was loaded into the van, Hawkins, ever affable, took the movers to lunch. During their absence someone conveniently stole the van. Hawkins silenced concerns with a peremptory wave of his hand. No big deal. It was all insured. The policy paid off to the tune of $109,000: Hawkins and Hanson were on their way.

They started a sportswear clothing chain called Just Sweats. The timing was perfect. Their Ohio-based business caught the eighties exercise wave and rode it to phenomenal success. In just over a year they went from a single shop to twenty-two outlets with annual sales in excess of $8.5 million.

But by 1986 they were bored, and running a successful company took time, something both seemed woefully short of. Hawkins's restlessness found expression in a jet-set lifestyle of Porsches, drugs, beautiful people, frantic sex and hustle, hustle, hustle. Hanson, part patrician, part lover, moved at a slower but equally licentious pace. He was under no illusions. The young studs that he adored and bedded tolerated him only because he was rich. Now, if he only had more money . . .

This was where the third coconspirator came in. They needed his expertise to pull off the ultimate swindle. There was just one problem: they did not trust him. Speed freaks never inspire confidence and this man had a monster habit that had left him fly-blown, glassy-eyed and broke. Unlike Hanson and Hawkins, his career was on a giddy downward spiral. He had known the good life and thrown it away. Over the years, millions of dollars had skipped through his increasingly jittery fingers, mostly gone to fuel his hopeless addiction to methamphetamine, or crank, as it was commonly known. This craving for speed had cost him a marriage, his home, his business, all contact with the deeply religious sect that had welcomed him. He desperately needed to reclaim his place in the world. More than anything he needed money, fast. For that, he would do anything . . .

It hadn't always been that way. Back in his youth Richard Pryde Boggs had been a textbook example of the American dream at work—a Depression era kid who had dragged himself up by his bootstraps all the way to respected city elder and the kind of money and trappings that went with such status. It was an ascent often imagined, rarely achieved. Like most who make the climb, Boggs was blessed with an unflinching will to succeed and boundless charm. Add brains, as well, and he seemed unstoppable.

He began life in South Dakota, but spent most of his early childhood in Casper, Wyoming. Jobs and money were scarce and, with the Depression biting hard, the Boggs family joined the mass migration to Southern California in 1939. They settled in Glendale, a suburb of Los Angeles. Boggs attended the local high school until 1951, then studied at UCLA. Five years later he graduated at the top of his class with a degree in zoology.

His graduation coincided with America's strongest economic boom in decades. Fortunes awaited those with the right stuff. Boggs wasn't stupid. Zoology degrees looked

impressive framed on the wall but they didn't amount to
much in the job market. He knew where the big money lay.
America's medical profession was just taking its first ten-
tative steps away from the traditional calling-at-all-hours-
with-a-black-bag role of the doctor toward a corporate
approach. That, combined with recent major advances in
medicine and treatment, had served to elevate the previously underpaid general practitioner into a wealthy pillar
of society, feted and admired, often dangerously so. Now
if Boggs, who was hell-bent on being a part of that environment, could only raise the cash to attend medical
school . . .

Salvation came in the form of a generous Wyoming
friend who promised to underwrite his college expenses
for no other reason than that she admired the young man's
determination to succeed. He enrolled at the College of
Medical Evangelists, today called the Loma Linda Medical
School.* At the same time he converted to the Seventh Day
Adventist creed of abstinence from alcohol, tobacco and
meat. It was a transformation no less dramatic or whole-
hearted than that of Paul on the road to Damascus. Boggs
became a model of piety and rectitude. He was also an excellent student.

Nineteen sixty-one was a banner year. He not only qualified, but married Lola Cleveland, a mathematics teacher
who had also helped support him during his medical training. It was around this time that Boggs's peculiarly para-
doxical nature first revealed itself. Having meticulously
repaid the medical school obligation, he approached his
benefactor for another loan, this time to start up in practice.
She readily agreed. Boggs borrowed $31,000 and this time

*Curiously enough, another graduate of the Loma Linda Medical School
was Dr. Bernard Finch; see Chapter 10.

neglected to repay a penny. Even so, his charm pulled him through. The friend later said, "I don't care. He's a brilliant doctor and I think the world of him."

Going to work at the Los Angeles County General Hospital, Boggs made a big impression on his fellow physicians who smoothed his entry into the prestigious Boston City Hospital for further studies. In 1967 he returned to finish his neurology training in Los Angeles and was made head of the neurology department at the Rancho Los Amigos Hospital.

Nobody ever accused Boggs of being a shirker. He had a boundless capacity for hard work and, with it, came the kind of lifestyle he had always craved. He purchased a sprawling mock-Tudor mansion nestled in a fold of the Pasadena hills and set about converting it into a monument to himself. Visitors could admire the life-size portrait of Richard Boggs that dominated the living room fireplace; any lingering doubts they might have entertained were dispelled by the gleaming Rolls Royce Silver Wraith II parked in the drive. At weekends the backyard was filled with laughter and sun-drenched barbecues, usually attended by doctors and their families. Tall, powerfully built, Boggs moved languidly through the throng, confident and successful, dispensing bonhomie and steaks with equal facility.

But there were other, less likeable, facets to Boggs's character. He had a terrifying capacity for instant and unexpected rage, a practical joker one minute, arrogant nitpicker the next. And he could be cruel. Once, while he was teaching, a medical student inadvertently put on his rubber gloves backwards. In front of a full class, Boggs bore down on the hapless student and forced him to repeat the procedure ten times, reveling in the young man's humiliation. Outside work hours he could be equally unpredictable. At a wedding, when the minister asked if there was anyone present who had any reason why the couple should not be married, Boggs jumped to his feet in mock protest. Only Boggs seemed able to find any humor in the incident; everyone else was appalled.

But most saw the Richard Boggs that he wanted the world to see: charming, witty in conversation, a man who cherished art and music, always ready to pick up the bill when dining with friends, trusting, some said, to the point of naïveté.

With his life on a seemingly endless upward curve, he never ceased casting around for ways to rise above the crowd. Vaulting ambition and unadulterated success have ways of dimming perspective and Boggs was no exception to the rule. In 1970 he came up with a revolutionary plan to provide health care for as many as 100,000 patients. A great talker, he convinced a group of investors of the idea's economic feasibility, and incorporated an operation called Satellite Health Systems. Decades ahead of its time, at first the health maintenance organization worked like clockwork—twenty-two contract doctors, working from a single building in Hollywood, provided medical care for more than 25,000 patients. Stories of Satellite's success spread like wildfire, all the way to the White House. Boggs had been recognized as a shining beacon of capitalism with a heart and, as such, deserving of a phone call from the president. When Richard Nixon came on the line, Boggs proudly listened as his groundbreaking success received praise from the highest office in the land.

But it was all a sham: the numbers just weren't there. By 1974 the large overheads and small membership sent Satellite into a tailspin. The dream shattered. Boggs, broke and bitter, had no alternative but to declare bankruptcy. Relatives and acquaintances agreed that it was this failure that unhinged him. As one patient put it, "We just saw him disintegrate."

Over the next two years his bills multiplied into millions; he owed the government, banks, leasing agencies, countless friends, everyone. Things became so bad that he could not keep up his American Medical Association membership. Nonpayment of dues also resulted in expulsion from the American Neurological Association. As his financial woes mounted, Boggs went on a borrowing binge. A fellow physician lent him $14,000 to satisfy the IRS; Boggs welshed on the loan. Only court action enabled the erstwhile friend to get his money back.

His work also deteriorated. Years later an official at a hospital where Boggs had privileges remembered: "He showed us that he really wasn't interested in our plans. That was a terrible disappointment. We thought he was very bright, but he was always looking for the easy way out . . . I was glad when he finally up and quit one day. We didn't have to fire him." Two other hospitals weren't so charitable. In 1976 both Glendale Memorial Hospital and Verdugo Hills Hospital quietly released Boggs from their staff for undisclosed disciplinary reasons.

This era highlights one of the more unsavory episodes of Richard Boggs's decline. Despite losing his privileges at three Glendale area hospitals, not once was he reported to the California Medical Board (CMB). The same system that kept fellow arch-incompetent Charles Friedgood* in practice now worked to salvage Boggs's career.

In order to make good on his losses he practiced medicine at a breakneck pace, very often starting his day at 5:00 AM, making rounds or assisting a neurosurgeon in surgery, then rushing back to his office or from one hospital to an-

*See chapter 2.

other, often not returning home until eleven or twelve o'clock that night. It was a backbreaking schedule, one no doctor could keep up indefinitely. Even Boggs, a bull of a man, grew frazzled, worn-out. In desperation he turned to chemically induced stamina.

Amphetamines—or speed—are insidious drugs. Like most addictives they require incremental doses to maintain the same effect. The downside is wicked. Massive mood-swings, coupled with bottomless bouts of depression and paranoia, often lead to irreversible personality changes. When Boggs began snorting crank, a form of methamphet-amine, at first he loved it—the boundless energy, the clar-ity of thought. But as his intake ballooned, he became wild-eyed, hyperactive, the victim of endless conspiracies, or so he thought. To guard against these dangers, both real and imagined, he began carrying a gun and boasting of im-portant Mafia connections. Acquaintances did not know whether to pity or despise him; most just looked the other way.

In 1978, with his life in a terrifying free fall, Boggs suf-fered another reversal. Unable to cope with her husband's increasingly irrational behavior, Lola left him. The breakup brought more than release from an unhappy mar-riage, it allowed Boggs, at last, to admit the duality in his sexual nature. It had always been there, a yearning for young studs and rough sex; now he was free to indulge those appetites without check. He began frequenting Hollywood's gay bars, cranked up and ready to pay for any kind of sex available.

At one hundred dollars a trick, such habits did not come cheap. In 1981 Lola had to sue Boggs to collect $33,000 in unpaid child support, despite the fact that his income for the year was $155,000. She also told the court that Boggs had threatened to kill her on several occasions, once boasting, "I could hire someone to snuff you."

That same year Boggs was finally reported to the CMB. Following the death of a patient from a drug overdose, the Glendale Adventist Medical Center, in a letter to the board, cited "extensive evidence of patient harm, patient suffering."

Still, no investigation was made. Boggs continued to practice medicine, running so-called "sleep clinics" for people with sleep disorders. More of a subterfuge than a clinic, the scheme allowed Boggs access to closely regulated sedatives, the kind that were popular but difficult to acquire on the street. Word got around and soon reached the ear of a teenage fitness enthusiast named John Hawkins.

Like almost everyone else who met Hawkins, Boggs fell completely under the young man's spell. When Hawkins flashed that smile and asked for quaaludes and other marketable drugs, the doctor was powerless to refuse. It was the same story with steroids which the narcissistic young bodybuilder used to inflate his frame to even more impossible dimensions.

Boggs's reputation for "loose scrips"—someone prepared to prescribe any amount of drugs if the price was right—made him a household name in the bars and among Hollywood junkies. Whatever you wanted, Boggs could deliver. In 1983 his recklessness again caught up with him when yet another patient died from a drug overdose. This time the CMB did investigate. Evidence showed that "patients were coming almost one hundred miles to his office" to receive prescriptions for addictive drugs. The doctor appointed by the CMB to head the investigation found that three patients had died in five years. His report concluded,

"Dr. Boggs appears to have made a habit of supplying dangerous, habituating drugs to drug addicts. His medical care contributed to the death of each of these patients."

Anyone expecting that Boggs's medical license would be automatically canceled after such conclusions was sorely mistaken. Again the CMB neglected to act. Boggs kept on writing scrips for anyone who had the money. He needed to. His finances were in a shambles. Litigation had stacked up over $1 million in uncollectable debts through sixty liens and judgments. Collectors dogged his footsteps. They garnished his office receipts, repossessed his furniture and office equipment. County marshals tried to sequester his Rolls Royce. The IRS even slapped a padlock on his office for default on back taxes.

Boggs responded by opening up another office across the street. And it was from there, at 7:04 AM on April 16, 1988, that a 911 call was made to the Glendale emergency services. Dr. Boggs sounded anxious. He needed assistance immediately. A patient, complaining of chest pains, had collapsed. Paramedics rushed over but were too late—the patient lay dead on the floor. Although there was nothing untoward, procedural policy in such situations dictated that the police be notified. Two officers were despatched to the scene. Neither was expecting anything out of the ordinary.

Just a routine call.

They were met by Dr. Boggs. Both thought him somewhat disheveled for a physician but put that down to the early hour and the circumstances. He showed them the dead man lying in the surgery. Boggs identified him as Melvin Eugene Hanson, an Ohio-based businessman who frequently came to Los Angeles on buying trips. Boggs told how Hanson had left a message on his answering machine at approximately 3:30 AM, saying he had been drinking and was now suffering shortness of breath and chest pain. Could the doctor see him right away? Boggs, aware of Hanson's long-standing heart condition, set off for his surgery as soon as he received the message.

He arrived at 5:00 AM to find Hanson waiting for him. After a preliminary examination, Boggs ran an electrocardiogram. Once the test was complete, Boggs went into his office to write up the results, leaving Hanson in the surgery. Suddenly he heard a loud thud. Boggs ran back and found that Hanson had collapsed, an apparent heart attack victim. After attempting unsuccessfully to revive Hanson, Boggs dialed 911 but the line was busy. He resumed artificial respiration and kept at it for forty-five minutes, then tried calling 911 again. This time he got through.

On the surface it sounded like a routine incident, just one more life cut tragically short by heart disease, soon forgotten about, and ninety-nine times out of a hundred that would have been the end of it. But on this occasion fate played a hand—both the police officers had some medical background. Patrolman Timothy Spruill had married a nurse, while his partner, Jim Lowry, was the son of a cardiologist. Instinctively they felt uneasy. Several factors did not add up. From their own observations, both reckoned that the corpse had been dead much longer than the two hours that Boggs claimed; then there was Boggs's insistence that the 911 number had been busy at 6:00 AM, not normally a hectic time for emergency calls. That could be checked out later, but what really created suspicion was that the time-stamped EKG tape Boggs claimed he ran at five o'clock, actually registered 12:02 AM This left only three options: the machine was faulty; Boggs, in all the confusion, had made a mistake; or he was lying. Both officers suspected the latter.

And there was something else. Apart from the usual collection of credit cards and the like, Hanson's wallet contained a photocopy of his birth certificate. Spruill and Lowry exchanged glances. How many people carry around a copy of their own birth certificate? It all seemed too pat, too convenient.

A check of Hanson's medical records, which Boggs had on file, revealed blue eyes, brown hair, 155 lbs., all details which tallied with the corpse, except maybe the weight. The dead man seemed a little heavier, but weight was always such a variable, a few pounds here or there didn't mean a thing. Nevertheless, the two officers took the unusual step of requesting a lab technician to photograph the body. They also asked for fingerprints. Just in case . . .

After the body was removed to the medical examiner's office, Spruill and Lowry briefed Detective Jim Peterson about their suspicions. For reasons which would later become apparent, Peterson asked the pathologists to look for evidence of sexual assault. They found none. In fact, they didn't find much of anything, except that Hanson's bloodstream was flooded with alcohol. Minus any sign of foul play and prompted by Dr. Boggs's diagnosis, the medical examiner recorded the cause of death as heart failure. Upon receipt of the report, Peterson ordered the case closed, even though just days earlier the Glendale Police Department had received a bizarre and possibly sinister complaint about this very same doctor.

A computer operator named Barry Pomeroy had come to them with a tale of being picked up at a West Hollywood bar in late March by a man calling himself Peter Richards. After a late-night meal, the two had visited Richards's office which was adorned with medical diplomas. Pomeroy couldn't help noticing that all the diplomas were in the name of Richard Pryde Boggs. When he pointed this out,

Richards smiled easily and told him that Boggs was his partner. Pomeroy accepted this and the rest of the evening passed without incident. Five days later Richards phoned Pomeroy and asked him out. Pomeroy agreed. Again they were at the office when, out of the blue, Richards suddenly asked Pomeroy if he would like an EKG exam. Pomeroy, unsure what to think, agreed. Seconds later Richards approached Pomeroy, arms spread wide as if to embrace him. Pomeroy readied himself for the expected amorous advance, only to feel a violent pain on the side of his neck. The shock sent him reeling. Only when his head cleared did he realize that Boggs was clutching a stun gun and had zapped him with it.

"It dawned on me that this man was trying to kill me," he said later. Richards kept jabbing with the gun. Pomeroy kept fighting him off. Eventually he knocked the gun from Richards's hand to the floor, The retaliation seemed to bring Richards to his senses. He began apologizing profusely, complained of having been under a lot of pressure lately, and promised to seek professional help. Pomeroy, who appears to have been remarkably trusting, allowed Richards to dress his wounds and drive him home.

There he began puzzling over the incident. Something did not smell right. Convinced that Richards was actually Richard Boggs, Pomeroy notified the Glendale police on April 9. They received the news cooly, convinced that this had all the hallmarks of another lovers' tiff; they actively dissuaded Pomeroy from pursuing the complaint. What Pomeroy did not know was that Dr. Boggs's brother, William, was an ex-Glendale police officer. Whether this had any bearing on departmental reluctance to investigate the doctor is unknown.

One week later, not even the discovery of a body in Boggs's surgery prompted any great official concern.

Peterson, leafing through Hanson's medical record, contacted the next of kin, John Hawkins in Columbus, and asked if Hanson and Boggs had been emotionally attached. Hawkins was askance. When Peterson hung up he decided that the Boggs/Pomeroy stun-gun episode and this latest incident were unconnected. The former he put down to merely another isolated outpouring of homosexual affection. He wasn't surprised. In Los Angeles, anything was possible . . .

Without intending this, Peterson's phone call set the ball rolling. That same afternoon Hawkins flew into Los Angeles from Ohio. After claiming Melvin Hanson's body, he whisked it to a nearby funeral home where it was cremated with a minimum of fuss or delay. Next, Hawkins dug out Hanson's life insurance policies, all of which named himself as sole beneficiary, and presented claims to three companies, totaling $1.5 million. To expedite the claims, he hired several lawyers, telling them that he needed the money urgently to prop up his now ailing company.

He wasn't exaggerating. Three months previous an audit of Just Sweats's finances had revealed some horrible deficiencies. As far as accountants could make out, Hanson had been taking advantage of Hawkins's frequent absences from the company to bleed it dry of funds. Almost $2 million had gone missing, as had Hanson. Hawkins, furious at being robbed, swore he would track Hanson down. This he did, running his erstwhile partner to ground in Los Angeles, only to learn that Hanson was in the terminal stages of heart disease. Hawkins flew back to Columbus and sadly informed employees at Just Sweats of Hanson's tragic condition. He also advised them that he had purchased Hanson's share in the company and would now do everything possible to restore the company to a sound financial footing. For the past three months he had attempted to do just that, without any noticeable improvement. At the time of Hanson's death, Just Sweats was barely solvent.

Desperate for cash, Hawkins kept hounding the insurance companies for payment. The pressure paid off. On July 7 Farmers Insurance relented and mailed Hawkins a check for $1 million. His intentions soon became clear. Far from using the funds to plug his leaky company, he used them to finance a wild orgy of sex and drugs. Even by Hawkins's own record-breaking standards it was one hell of a bash. His splurge might have been a little less exuberant had he known that doubts were already beginning to surface about the legitimacy of his claim.

As early as June, insurance investigators had contacted the Glendale police, anxious to confirm that the body was that of Melvin Hanson. Peterson promised to obtain a copy of Hanson's driver's license. But, as the bureaucratic wheels creaked ever more slowly and Hawkins's lawyers kept clamoring for payment, Farmers Insurance had no alternative but to settle the claim. Just six days later, Peterson received a copy of Hanson's 1985 California driver's license.

Neither the photograph nor the thumbprint matched those of the body in Dr. Boggs's office.

No one likes to think that they've been conned. And in this instance, as often happens, official embarrassment was countered with a blur of official activity. Confronted by irrefutable evidence that the dead body was not Melvin Hanson, the coroner's office revised their findings to show cause of death as "undetermined." A reexamination of various fluids taken from the body crushed any lingering suspicion that this was Melvin Hanson.

The dead man was infected with full-blown AIDS. Hanson's records showed that, shortly before his "death," he had tested HIV negative.

Establishing who the dead person was not proved markedly easier than giving him a name. Every city morgue has its share of bodies, unnamed except for a tag on the big toe that says either John or Jane Doe. In vast transit camps like Los Angeles, people of all ages drift in and out daily, without family or relatives to record their movements. When they die most get lost in the shuffle. On this occasion, however, the Glendale Police Department was lucky. In September a call from the US Department of Justice revealed that the deceased's thumbprint matched an April missing persons report. Bearing the photo taken at Boggs's surgery, detectives called on the elderly Hollywood woman who had filed the report on her missing nephew. Cleo Fasulo studied the photo for a moment, then sadly nodded her head.

Ellis Henry Greene had been found.

Convinced by now that they were dealing with a major insurance fraud at least, and probably much worse, the police put out a wanted bulletin on Melvin Hanson. In the meantime they began looking long and hard at the enigmatic Dr. Boggs.

He professed amazement when told that the dead man was not Hanson. The idea was preposterous, he said, why should Ellis Greene have pretended to be Melvin Hanson for seven years? The police, unimpressed either by Boggs's reasoning or his loud denials of culpability, continued digging.

They learned from a woman, who had worked as Boggs's receptionist for fifteen years, of repeated phone calls from pharmacists, querying the frequency and amount of his prescriptions. Taken in conjunction with earlier reports of blatant overprescribing, this led investigators to conclude that, for years, Richard Boggs had been a high-level drug dealer. Verification came at his office where detectives discovered all the paraphernalia necessary for the manufacture of top-grade methamphetamine. Most of this he sold; the remainder he either used himself or traded for sex.

Even so, none of this proved murder and none of it proved that Boggs was party to any insurance swindle. For that, the police needed stronger evidence. Help was just a few months away.

On January 29, 1989 a nervous-looking tourist wearing scarlet shorts, a yellow shirt and tennis shoes was stopped for questioning at Dallas-Fort Worth International Airport. Beneath the edgy expression his face had a taut, unnatural look, as if he had recently undergone cosmetic surgery. He had just arrived from Acapulco and gave his name as Wolfgang von Snowden. When customs officials went through his luggage they found $14,000 in cash hidden in the lining as well as identification papers under numerous pseudonyms. One name in particular stood out—Ellis Greene. There was also a book entitled *How to Create a New Identity.*

Despite the plastic surgery, Melvin Hanson made no serious attempt to deny his identity. On the contrary, he seemed relieved. His only plea, prior to being returned to Ohio on embezzlement and insurance fraud charges, was that he be housed in the homosexual section of Tarrant County Jail in Fort Worth. The request was granted.

Investigators learned that Hanson had embarked on his new identity as Wolfgang von Snowden (which he seems to have had trouble in spelling) two months before his "death." They also discovered that he had signed a rental agreement for a Miami apartment using the nom de plume of Wolfgang Eugene *Vonsnowden*. For character references he gave two names: John Hawkins was one, the other . . . Dr. Richard Boggs.

With the connection made, events moved quickly. Telephone records showed a flurry of activity between Boggs, Hanson and Hawkins during the months leading up to Hanson's connived death. Moreover, on April 15, 1988—the day of Ellis Greene's disappearance—Hanson had flown from Miami to Los Angeles and checked in at the Holiday Inn in Glendale, just three blocks from Boggs's office, under the name of Wolfgang Vonsnowden. During the next afternoon he had taken a flight back to Miami, then south to Key West where he opened a sizeable bank account in the name of Ellis Henry Greene. Throughout this period he continued to stay in touch with Boggs and Hawkins by phone.

An examination of Boggs's bank statements revealed that, in May 1988, he had received an unexplained check for $6,500 from Hawkins. Detectives decided it was time to have a word with the doctor.

On February 3, 1989 Dr. Richard Boggs's precipitous slide from grace hit rock bottom. He was in the midst of clearing out his possessions from his office suite, having just been evicted for nonpayment of rent, when detectives arrived to arrest him. At the DA's office, Boggs was charged with nine counts of murder, conspiracy and insurance fraud and held without bail.

With two of the three suspects in custody, all that was needed now was to find John Hawkins. That proved easier said than done. The only clue to his whereabouts was his Mercedes convertible found abandoned at Columbus airport. He obviously was not short of funds. Between them, Hanson and Hawkins had plundered $1.8 million from Just Sweats. Together with the insurance payout Hawkins had working capital of almost $3 million. For several months he dodged around the US, staying with numerous girlfriends, breaking hearts, breaking promises, then he slipped from view. Sightings came in from as far afield as Florida and California, then petered out entirely—John Barrett Hawkins, the hustler supreme, had vanished.

He left behind him a fragmented prosecution. As the trial date approached, hopes of trying Boggs and Hanson together faded. It would have to be Boggs or nothing.

At his trial, Richard Boggs was portrayed as the mastermind behind the almost perfect crime. Whether he originated the murderous plan is debatable; Hanson and Hawkins were both old hands when it came to defrauding insurance companies, but certainly the scheme could not have worked without the doctor's active support.

The prosecution alleged that Boggs had first incapacitated Greene with a stun gun and then smothered him, an idea stridently contested by the defense. They maintained that no murder had taken place. Yes, their client was "unquestionably guilty" of conspiring to swindle insurance benefits by falsely substituting Ellis Greene's identity for that of Melvin Hanson, but defense attorney Dale Rubin insisted that the object was money, not murder. The body, he said, had come from a local morgue.

Boggs listened with mild distaste. Throughout the trial he sat slumped over the defense table, doodling and infrequently looking up. The only time he evinced any real interest in the proceedings was when Melvin Hanson appeared, to prove to the jurors that he was still alive. All Hanson did was show up; he steadfastly refused to give evidence against his friend.

After two days of deliberation the jury convicted Boggs of first degree murder and eight other counts of insurance fraud. Prosecution hopes of strapping Boggs into the gas chamber received a severe setback during the trial's penalty phase when two women jurors refused to recommend the death penalty. Their recalcitrance resulted in a mistrial. Three months later a second jury also refused to sentence Boggs to death and he was imprisoned for life. The doctor did not seem to care either way, having learned just before the trial that he was infected with the AIDS virus.

In August 1991, John Hawkins's three-year flight from justice ended in Caligari, Sardinia, when agents from the U.S. Naval Investigative Service arrested the young playboy aboard his red catamaran, *Carpe Diem*. Hawkins had been living the kind of life he'd always lusted after, cruising the Mediterranean with a bevy of girls and the occasional young hunk, indulging every kind of sexual nuance imaginable. His capture highlights the way communications have shrunk the planet to the global village foreseen by media guru Marshall McCluhan. An installment of *The Oprah Winfrey Show* featuring the Boggs case had been shown on Italian television. A young woman—Hawkins's most recent conquest—had watched the show in a blind rage. Her fury stemmed from the fact that Hawkins had given no hint of his bisexuality; she found that unforgivable and informed the authorities.

To change his appearance Hawkins had undergone chin implants and collagen lip injections. But there was nothing he could do about a rare skin condition that left him with a lack of skin pigmentation in his penis. Even without the fingerprint evidence, this would have been sufficient to identify him. For two years he languished in an Italian prison, fighting extradition. Once he escaped but was recaptured in the prison grounds. To secure Italian cooperation, the American authorities had to promise that they would not seek the death penalty. In July 1992, John Barrett Hawkins was returned to the US.

After considerable legal wrangling, on March 21, 1995, Hanson and Hawkins stood trial in Los Angeles for murder and various other charges. Both admitted the insurance scam, but denied all knowledge of the murder. Their only crime, they said, was to pay Boggs $50,000 to steal a corpse from a hospital or morgue. On August 8, 1995, both men were convicted of conspiracy to commit murder, grand theft and an additional count of fraud. The following day, the jury found Hanson guilty of murder. Because the jury deadlocked on the murder charge against Hawkins, a mistrial was declared. With the case getting messier by the minute, the district attorney's office decided to cut its losses and threw out the murder charge against Hawkins. On October 13, 1995, he was sentenced to twenty-five years to life. One month earlier, Hanson was given life without parole.

Had it not been for the inquisitiveness of two patrolmen, the murder of Ellis Greene might have gone unrecorded and unpunished. Having said that, the remarkably slipshod tactics employed by the conspirators in the crime's aftermath suggest that their own stupidity would have brought the murder to light. And there was always the possibility that such a profitable exercise would have spawned a duplicate. (Hawkins, apparently, was already arranging his own "death" when this particular scheme unraveled.) The rewards were just too great. Melvin Hanson knew that. When asked, following his arrest, if he could come up with bail of $5 million, the larcenous salesman gave it a few moments' thought, then remarked slyly, "If they let me die a few more times, I can."

13. THE HALLOWEEN TRICKSTER

For more than four decades the city of Boston has had to wrestle with the uncomfortable knowledge that it spawned the world's very first made-for-TV serial killer. At the beginning of the sixties, habitual homicide was nothing new for America—as much as four decades earlier, the likes of Carl Panzram and Earle Nelson had shown just what was possible when the career killer really applies himself—but they were traveling psychopaths and those were quieter times. Broadly speaking, their outrages were newsworthy only in those localities affected. By the second half of the twentieth century, all that had changed. Television's steamroller advance meant that details of sensational murders could now be pumped almost instantly into living rooms from Maine to California. In a stroke of quite exquisite serendipity, a bizarre string of killings that terrified New Englanders in the early sixties was ideally timed to take advantage of this transition. Between June 1962 and January 1964, thirteen women, mostly middle-aged or elderly, were strangled in their homes in the Boston area.

The slayings were spectacularly gruesome, and while some members of the investigative task force privately doubted that they were the work of just one man, so far as the TV crews, newspaper and radio reporters were concerned, it was simply too good an opportunity to miss. Latching on to the notion of a city in panic, they marketed the "Boston Strangler" with a Madison Avenue–like ferocity and thoroughness. Little wonder, then, that the media coverage that first straddled America and then girdled the globe, followed by an exhaustive book and a popular movie, was sufficient to guarantee the Boston Strangler's induction into the Murderer's hall of infamy, alongside the likes of Jack the Ripper and the Zodiac Killer.

With the capture and incarceration of Albert DeSalvo—a lifelong sex offender who admitted the killings but was never charged—the people of Boston heaved a collective sigh of relief. Most assumed that the worst was over and struggled to put the crimes behind them. In November 1973, that relieved sigh increased by a few decibels when one of DeSalvo's fellow inmates took a knife to the self-confessed strangler. With his death, the final chapter seemed to have closed on this dreadful saga.

In common with every major US city, Boston continued to host its share of murders, but for the most part it was the usual run-of-the mill mix of domestics and drugs, ghastly for those involved, of little interest to those unaffected. Happily, the city remained free from the modern curse of the serial killer. But in the fall of 1999, more than a few residents of Norfolk County, a lush and leafy district just to the southwest of Boston, had reason to wonder if the ghost of Albert DeSalvo had been resurrected.

The first killing took place on the morning of December 1, 1998. At just after eight o'clock, longtime Walpole residents Thomas and Irene Kennedy had gone walking in the town's beautiful Bird Park, as they had most mornings for the previous ten years. As was also their custom, they agreed to split up and reunite in thirty minutes. When Irene, age seventy-five, failed to show at the designated meeting place, her worried husband went off in search. At 8:50 AM he found her. She was lying in the woods about five feet from a gravel path. She had been stabbed more than two dozen times, throttled and then sexually mutilated. The sickening nature of the attack, magnified by its scarcity—statistics show that, crimewise, Norfolk County is one of the safest places in America—sparked a knee-jerk reaction from the law enforcement agencies involved. In quick order, a local man was arrested, charged with murder, held for several weeks, then released. There were large portions of humble pie all round as embarrassed investigators faced the media and shamefacedly admitted that they had nabbed the wrong guy. Compounding their humiliation was the total absence of an alternative suspect.

An uneasy peace settled over Walpole, with everyone praying that the Kennedy killing was an isolated aberration that would darken memories and nothing else. They wanted the killer caught of course, but most of all they wanted their peace of mind restored. And for several months they got their wish. Then tragedy struck again.

The historic town of Westwood is rightly proud of its impressive eighteenth century architecture and glorious fall foliage, and lies just seven miles north of Walpole. It had been home to Richard Reyenger for almost half his life. Nowadays, the eighty-two-year-old retired woodworker liked nothing better than getting up at dawn to chase the bass and trout in nearby Buckmaster Pond. Most days he did okay. But on August 21, 1999, his luck ran out for good. He was found at 7:40 AM, prone on the shoreline, unconscious and bleeding from a disastrous head wound. (It was later determined that he had been felled with a single ax blow that sliced five inches deep into his skull.) He died in the hospital without recovering consciousness.

The fact that, just a few miles and a matter of months apart, two elderly people had been bludgeoned to death while taking early morning walks in a public park was bound to spark fears of a serial killer. Even police spokespersons conceded the possibility. It was the sheer senselessness of the killings that baffled everyone. That, and the maddening lack of suspects.

As summer faded into fall, with no obvious name in the frame, some investigators began thinking the unthinkable: if there really was a "Park Killer," then their best chances of nailing him would come only if he struck again. They didn't have long to wait.

Some twelve miles north of Westwood lies the town of Wellesley. Besides being home to one of the most prestigious girls' schools in America, this pastoral outpost on the Charles River is an upmarket haven of tranquility and peace, a magnet for intellectuals and businesspeople alike. The writers Sylvia Plath and Vladimir Nabokov have both called it home, and with a median family income three times the national average, Wellesley is the kind of place where successful people come to raise families, mix with their social peers, and soak up the rustic splendor. Serious crime was almost unheard of. Locals had to really stretch their memories to recall the last murder hereabouts, back in 1969 when a young woman was shot and killed by a jilted lover. So, Wellesley was the last place that anyone would expect a serial killer to strike.

Until Halloween 1999.

Mabel Greineder was just fifty-eight years old when she left her split-level home on Cleveland Road in Wellesley on the last morning of her life. She had much to be thankful for. Her husband Dirk was a world-renowned allergist, they had raised three great kids, all of whom had attended Yale and just recently Mabel—or May, as most people knew her—had been hitting the books hard, intent on reviving her former career as a nurse practitioner. No, life couldn't have been better, even on a dank, foggy morning like this, as she and Dirk herded one of their two German shepherds—the other was experiencing psychological problems and remained at home, sedated on Prozac—into the minivan for the half-mile drive to Morse's Pond.

Besides providing Wellesley with its drinking water, Morse's Pond acts as unofficial town playground. In the summer, locals make the most of its sandy beach and surrounding woods. When the bitter New England winter begins to bite, it's the turn of the ice skaters to commandeer the frozen lake. At over one hundred acres, the park is large and crisscrossed with hiking trails that weave in and out of the pine, oak and maple trees. The Greineders came here most days to exercise their dogs.

This morning, though, they had only been walking for a few minutes when Mabel stumbled on a stone and wrenched her back. Rather than spoil her husband's enjoyment, she selflessly insisted that Greineder carry on without her. They agreed to rendezvous at a landmark rock that stood on the park's main access road. After satisfying himself that Mabel was all right, Greineder hitched up his red backpack and, within seconds, he and Zephyr were swallowed up by the thick woods as they headed for Old Beach. They were gone about ten minutes.

It was getting close to nine o'clock when Greineder started back to the prearranged meeting place. His journey took him through some of the most heavily wooded reaches of the park. Suddenly he jolted to a standstill. Blocking his path was a blood-drenched body.

Mabel lay motionless, her head caved in, throat slashed wide open. Her blouse had been pulled up and her pants pulled down.

Instinctively, Greineder ran forward and checked for a pulse in Mabel's neck. Nothing. In a reflex action he reached for his cell phone, only to realize it was back in the minivan. Frantic and panic-stricken, he turned and ran for assistance.

He had only covered a few yards when he spotted someone else out walking his dog. Greineder rushed up and asked the stranger if he had a phone. When William Kear said no, Greineder pointed behind him and blurted out that his wife "had been attacked," before dashing off to where his van was parked. A quarter mile later, out of breath and panting, he grabbed his cell phone.

The emergency call was logged at 8:56 AM.

"Help! I'm at the pond!" he yelled. "Someone attacked my wife!"

Wellesley police dispatcher Shannon Parillo was used to dealing with overwrought callers, but Greineder was in a dreadful state, barely coherent, and she struggled to unravel his labyrinthine pleas. Her first impression was that the caller's daughter had been attacked. Only after a considerable effort was she able to clarify the victim's identity.

"Is she injured?" Parillo asked.

"I think she's dead," Greineder said. "It's definitely an attack."

Asked by the dispatcher if he was with his wife, Greineder replied, "No, no, I'm way out. I had to go out to call you . . . I tried to see if there was anything to do," adding later, "There's nothing I can do . . . I think she's dead. I'm not sure. I'm a doctor . . . she looks terrible."

Parillo told him to stay calm and promised that someone would be with him as soon as possible.

Just minutes later Patrolman Paul J. Fitzpatrick roared into the park. Greineder flagged him down and guided him to where the body lay, all the while explaining how he and Mabel had become separated, and how he had returned to find her dead. When they reached the body, he dropped to his knees, overcome by grief, and cried out, "This is my wife! Who could have done this to my wife?"

He made a pitiable sight, blood streaks all over him, across the sleeves of his yellow windbreaker, down the black jeans, and onto his white Reeboks. Fitzpatrick had been on the force for twenty-eight years, but nothing in his experience or the training manual had taught him how to comfort a husband who'd just found his wife butchered like a hog.

Within minutes the park was full of sirens and emergency personnel. Local, state, and Massachusetts Bay Transit Authority police worked as a coordinated team, while divers probed the depths of Morse's Pond. Even though the park was sealed off, it failed to prevent news of the murder spreading like wildfire through the local community. Few who heard the gory details were in any doubt—the "Park Killer" had struck again.

The similarities were undeniable: an older than average victim, murdered in the early morning, in a remote park setting. The killing of Mabel Greineder brought one other coincidence to the mix. Like the first victim, Irene Kennedy, she too had been out walking with her husband, only to become separated. Did this mean that the killer was out there stalking couples, waiting his opportunity to strike? By nightfall the chain of coincidences had been stretched to the breaking point, with some of the more fanciful imaginations zeroing in on the fact that all the killings had occurred in towns beginning with the letter *W.* This was just too surreal. A killer who selected his victims through a gazetteer?

For the rest of that day, Greineder remained at the Wellesley police station, helping the officers with their inquiries. Eventually they accompanied him to the big house on Cleveland Road where he and Mabel had lived for twenty-four years. He seemed utterly broken, a man trapped in a vortex of human disintegration. The police stayed with him for hours, asking questions, as they have to, requesting items of his clothes for routine analysis. But after they left and the darkness closed in around him, Dr. Dirk Greineder struggled to come to terms with his utter desolation. He didn't pray, because that wasn't his way. Nor did he seek the comfort of his three children. No, the tall, bespectacled pillar of the local community had another, rather more original method of working through the grief. He phoned a hooker.

Of all the doctors profiled within these pages, German-born Dirk Greineder was probably the most brilliant, certainly the most privileged. In 1942, while he was still a toddler, his parents managed to escape the madness of Hitler's Reich and make their way to Lebanon, where his father, a physician, landed a job teaching at the American University of Beirut. Beirut in the 1950s offered a glitzy, sophisticated lifestyle, where diplomats, wealthy arms dealers, intellectuals and spies brushed up against each other at cocktail parties, exchanging witty conversation and the occasional nugget of intelligence. Young Dirk soaked up the atmosphere like a sponge. He also raced impatiently through his classes. His family decided that his education should be continued abroad, and after he obtained his high school diploma at the American

Community School, they immigrated to the United States. While it's true that Greineder enjoyed all the advantages that wealth and social influence could bring, he was light years away from being some feckless silver spooner. He was smart, very smart, fluent in four languages—German, English, French and Arabic—and bright enough to be accepted at Yale, where he majored in chemistry. Maddeningly for those less gifted, he even found time to double up as a jock, captaining the swim team and rowing with the varsity crew. But always the books came first. Given his pedigree, his career choice was entirely predictable. After graduating from Yale in 1962 he headed for Case Western Reserve University in Cleveland, Ohio, to study medicine. That was where he met Mabel. A year younger than Dirk, Mabel combined a fine intellect with dazzling good looks. After earning a degree in zoology at Hunter College in New York, she had come to Case Western to teach in the nursing program. The couple married in Cleveland on June 8, 1968, and moved to New York where Greineder did a two-year residency at Cornell Medical Center. Selflessly, Mabel put her own career aspirations on hold as she supported Dirk and raised a family.

Greineder's work as a post-doctoral researcher kept him out of Vietnam, and after a brief spell in Bethesda, Maryland, the Greineders moved to Wellesley in 1975. It wasn't long before Dirk was made an associate professor of medicine at Harvard Medical School.

Over the next two decades Greineder's career really took off. He was board certified in internal medicine and allergy and immunology, and his principal job was at Brigham and Women's Hospital, one of the nation's top research centers. One day a week he saw patients at the Harvard Vanguard Medical Associates office in Kenmore Square. It was a hectic schedule. Some reckoned his success came at a price. While marveling at his work ethic, they found him dour and joked that he must have undergone a humor bypass. If Greineder heard the chuckles behind his back, he didn't let on. His patients adored him and so long as the accolades kept on coming, he was content. And keep on coming they did. In 1997, he was cowinner of the Harvard Pilgrim Health Care Outstanding Physician Award. Two years later he published a study in *The Journal of Allergy and Clinical Immunology* that dealt with revised programs of pediatric asthma treatment. Contributions such as these made him one of the most highly regarded allergists in America.

If everything was outstanding at work, then Dirk Greineder's home life glowed like a Norman Rockwell painting. The children had come along at two-year intervals. Kirsten was the first in 1969, followed by Britt and Colin. They grew up with a father who served them fresh fruit every morning, drove them to swim meets, and coached their soccer teams. In time, all three kids would follow in their father's footsteps and attend Yale. Kirsten and Colin would take the family tradition one step further and each make medicine their life's work, while Britt entered the hurly-burly of the Boston business world.

Mabel, too, seemed fulfilled. She was active in her local church and in 1993, to help pay for Kirsten's medical tuition fees, she had taken a position as a nurse with her husband at Harvard Vanguard. She stayed for five years and then resigned. With Kirsten's upcoming marriage, Mabel had plenty to occupy her mind. Still, though, she entertained hopes of returning to nursing and was studying hard at the time of her death. Dirk, strongly supportive of this revived interest, was always on hand to help out with her term papers, either by checking facts or else typing footnotes.

To an awestruck world, Dirk and Mabel Greineder looked like a couple who had fallen asleep, dreamed their version of the American dream, then woken up to find it was reality. Only for it all to collapse in a blood-soaked heap on the morning of October 31, 1999.

Whoever killed Mabel Greineder had been brutally efficient. An autopsy performed by State Medical Examiner Stanton Kessler revealed the full extent of her injuries. She had been poleaxed with a blow to the rear of the head, possibly a hammer, then the killer had gone berserk with a knife. Kessler counted at least ten stab wounds, most to the back of the skull, but the lethal wound was a gaping 5½" by 2½" slash that ran from her left ear to the center of her throat. It sliced through her jugular vein, deep enough to strike the fifth vertebrae and sever the muscles that controlled her tongue. An absence of defensive wounds to the hands or arms told Kessler that Mabel was either struck down unexpectedly from behind, or knew her attacker. He also thought she had been dragged some distance after having fallen to the ground, judging from the scrape wounds on her back.

On one point Kessler was emphatic: such an attack would have produced copious amounts of blood, as Greineder had learned to his cost when he rushed to tend his stricken wife. Her blood was found all over him—except for the one place where it should have been.

State Trooper Martin Foley had been one of the first law enforcement officers on the scene, and like everyone else he had initially been struck by the similarities between this killing and the two previous slayings. But as he listened to Greineder's tearful account of how he had found his wife lying on the grass, then tried to lift her, a glaring discrepancy jumped out at him. He didn't beat about the bush.

"Did you wash your hands?" he asked Greineder point-blank.

"No."

"How do you explain the lack of blood on your hands?"

Greineder floundered for a second, and in the absence of any reasonable explanation or brilliant invention, muttered, "I can't." From this single observation—and Greineder's notably feeble response—was born the first doubt about his story.

Another anomaly had also come to light. When talking to Officer Fitzpatrick, who had accompanied him to the body, Greineder mentioned that his wife had twisted her back after stepping on a stone during their morning walk. A short time later he told Detective Jill Hogan that Mabel had hurt her back tossing a ball to their dog. It wasn't much, but it was an inconsistency, and as any experienced detective knows all too well, inconsistencies are the pebbles over which liars often trip.

Greineder was also acting suspiciously in other ways. Not only did he refuse to go to the medical examiner's office to view his wife's body, but he also forbade his children to attend as well, despite the fact that Kirsten, as a trainee doctor, was no stranger to violent trauma. By adhering to Greineder's wishes, his three children set the tone for an attitude that persists to the present day—unswerving support for their father.

In the meantime, crime scene investigators radiated outward from where the body had been found in their search for clues. Their sweep took them along a paved path south of the pond, through the woods, and ultimately to a storm drain. When Wellesley Police Sergeant Peter Nahass raised the lid and peered inside, his flashlight picked out an unnatural looking pile of leaves. Pushing the leaves to one side, he saw the blue handle of a two-pound Estwing hammer, a Schrade Old Timer folding knife with a four-inch blade, and a bloodstained right-handed brown work glove.

The location of this find was hugely significant. According to William Kear, when he'd first seen Greineder that morning, the doctor had been unaware of his presence, and had been striding along the access road before disappearing down this selfsame paved pathway. Kear lost sight of him for "no longer than twenty to thirty seconds." Only when Greineder reappeared did he run up to Kear, begging him for a cell phone.

After Greineder left, Kear had gone to investigate along the dirt path where Greineder said his wife lay. As he said later, "I saw some legs that were sticking out into the path." Kear stopped and peered fearfully about him. Perhaps the killer was still around. Maybe even watching him right now! With understandable trepidation, he retreated to what felt like a safer distance.

When queried about Kear's statement, Greineder freely admitted having been on the path where the weapons were found. He had, he claimed, caught sight of a "shadow or shadows" on this path, and, thinking that it might have been his wife's killer, had gone in pursuit. When he realized the futility of such a mission, he had about-faced and headed back. On his return journey he had bumped into Kear.

This raised yet another dichotomy. Because when the CSIs examined footprints left in the soil around Mabel's body, after eliminating themselves and everyone else associated with inquiry, only one set of prints remained; and these belonged to the victim's husband. If Greineder's story were true, this mystery assailant somehow managed to butcher Mabel and then dematerialize into the woods without leaving so much as a single footprint.

Piece by incriminating piece the evidence slotted together. One day later, another bloody glove—left-handed and an obvious match to the first glove—was discovered, this time in a storm drain just fifteen yards from where Greineder had parked his van. This meant that both gloves had been found in areas visited by Greineder.

As the appeal for witnesses gathered steam, yet another dog walker, Terence MacNally, came forward. He, too, had been at Morse's Pond on the morning of the murder, playing fetch with his dog, and between 8:40 and 8:50 AM, he had heard a "high-pitched yell," followed by several short, sharp cries. The noises had prompted MacNally's dog to scoot off into the woods, determined to root out the source of the disturbance. When MacNally had called, the dog came bounding back. As the woods fell silent once again, owner and dog continued on their walk, untroubled by the presence of anyone else and with nothing to explain those mysterious cries.

MacNally's story guided searchers to the area where his dog had gone briefly missing. There, beneath a thin layer of pine needles, they uncovered a strange cache of items: a pair of surgical gloves; two Ziploc bags; a bottle of lighter fluid; and an aluminum pan, the kind used to prepare meatloaf. All looked to have been hastily hidden. Perhaps, reasoned the investigators, the killer had been disturbed by MacNally or his dog, and, in his desperation to get away, had bungled his cleanup operation. Of course, the possibility existed that none of the items was connected to the murder of Mabel Greineder. All the same, it was puzzling.

When all the interviews were collated and cross-checked, one distinct conclusion could be drawn: four people had seen Dirk Greineder in the park that morning and yet none of these witnesses—all regular visitors to Morse's Pond—had spotted any strangers.

So far nothing had been found to deflect the focus of the

inquiry. As the district attorney's office subsequently admitted, right from the outset all investigative eyes were fixed very firmly in one direction and on just one suspect. Early press briefings reflected this conviction. Eager to allay public concerns, officers took the highly unusual step of stressing that the Halloween murder of Mabel Greineder was a discrete incident, wholly unrelated to the killings of Irene Kennedy and Richard Reyenger. One didn't need a PhD in cryptanalysis to unscramble the subtext and decipher the official belief that the killer was none other than Dirk Greineder.

When it comes to murder, investigative instincts are remarkably well honed; after all, homicide detectives deal with homicide suspects on a regular basis and quickly develop a nose for when someone is telling the truth. But nobody bats a thousand, and the appeals courts are littered with examples of how such a blinkered pursuit can backfire. It had happened right here in Norfolk County. Early on in the investigation of Irene Kennedy's murder, officers became convinced that a man named Edmund F. Burke was the killer and targeted all their efforts in this direction. He had been arrested and incarcerated for six weeks until being cleared by DNA analysis. The DA's office was desperate to avoid an embarrassing rerun of that fiasco.

In all fairness, though, when it came to Dirk Greineder, there was plenty to arouse suspicion. Take those scratches on the side of his neck, for instance. Interviewing officers had spotted them as they questioned Greineder just hours after the crime. Shaving mishaps, he explained unconvincingly. The doubts multiplied when, in a purely routine procedure, detectives asked if they might take his clothes for forensic examination. Greineder, who didn't quibble, stripped immediately, exposing a third scratch that ran across his chest. This he blamed on a rambunctious dog.

Officers leaned in more closely. So what about those dime-sized bruises on your left bicep? Greineder just shrugged. He had no idea where they'd come from.

It was also discovered that on the day before Mabel's death, Greineder had called into his local health club and requested that his membership be frozen immediately until February 2000. (Just two weeks after Mabel's death, he contacted the club again and filed for reactivation.)

When the full autopsy results on Mabel Greineder came back, they added to the thickening cloud of suspicion that shrouded her husband. Beneath her fingernails were fragments of skin, the kind often found when a victim has fought for life and scratched their assailant. Preliminary DNA analysis showed that these human cells came from someone other than the victim. A more exhaustive follow-up analysis showed that "someone" to be Dirk Greineder.

Greineder cast his mind back. Just before going to Morse's Pond on that fateful morning, he and Mabel had had sex. As part of the foreplay, Mabel had given him a backrub; this could well have resulted in his DNA being found under her fingernails.

So, the investigators wanted to know, how come your DNA also turned up on the knife and hammer?

Greineder remembered that before going to Morse's Pond, he and Mabel had suffered simultaneous nosebleeds and had shared a Kleenex. It was entirely possible, he explained with the authority born of a thousand consultations, that this action caused his DNA to be transferred to Mabel, and from there it migrated onto the murder weapons.

Simultaneous nosebleeds? In two mature adults? All leading to cross-contamination? As excuses go, this was smack in the middle of the "you gotta be kidding!" category, and served only to convince the detectives that their

decision to search Greineder's house as early as the night
of the crime had been entirely justified. What they'd already found had fueled their suspicions; what was yet to be
uncovered would strip away the veneer from Greineder's
marriage and expose it to the world as a crumbling sham.

First, they began with the family finances. Prosecutorial
eyes lit up like beacons when it was discovered that, on
October 29, just two days before Mabel was murdered, she
and Dirk had taken out $500,000 insurance policies on
each other's lives. Later, buried in the fine print, came the
deflating revelation that the policies had never actually
gone into effect, and that the beneficiaries were actually
the Greineder children, who would only inherit after the
death of both parents.

Setting that red herring aside, investigators still had
plenty to exercise their imaginations. Nine days after the
killing, Wellesley Police Chief Terrence Cunningham led a
search of Greineder's backyard and the doghouse that was
home to Zephyr and Wolf, the two German shepherds.
Inside the doghouse, Cunningham found a pair of brown
work gloves identical to those recovered from the crime
scene.

Another vital clue turned up inside the house. In the
pantry lay an opened box of heavy-duty one-gallon Ziploc
bags. There were seven remaining and, to the naked eye at
least, they looked indistinguishable from the two bags
found near Mabel's body. All the bags were sent to the FBI
Forensic Science Laboratory in Washington, DC for analysis.

Damaging as these discoveries undoubtedly were, the
investigators still felt hamstrung. They needed a motive.
Although not legally required to do so, every prosecutor
wants to be able to tell the jury, "The defendant carried out
this crime because . . ." And there seemed to be no earthly

reason why Dirk Greineder would want to murder his wife. Almost everyone the police spoke to described the Greineders as a loving, successful couple, with a great marriage and three wonderful kids. Only a couple of close acquaintances had misgivings. There was nothing that Ilsa Stark, Mabel's elder sister, could really put her finger on, but she'd always gained the impression that Dirk was very much the dominant partner in the relationship, and in recent years he'd become more withdrawn from the rest of the family. He'd missed the last four annual family vacations and when Mabel had needed money for some cosmetic surgery, it was Ilsa who footed the bill, not Dirk.

She also recalled one strange incident the day Mabel was killed. Ilsa and her daughter, Belinda Markel, had gathered with the Greineder family at their Wellesley home to mourn their loss. At one point Greineder took Belinda into his study and announced that he and Mabel had had sex that morning "but there was nothing wrong with that because they were married." Belinda looked askance. In all the years she had known Dirk she had never known him to be so forthright or explicit. When the police heard this, they too thought it sounded odd, and went back to reinterview Greineder. They asked if he was keeping something from them. The Harvard physician took a moment to consider his position. Then he unburdened himself.

His story about having had sex with Mabel on the morning of her murder was a lie, he said. In truth, they had not been sexually active for several years, because intercourse caused his wife pelvic pain and he had respected that condition. Understandably this admission raised a few investigative eyebrows, especially as there didn't seem to be any reason for the original fabrication. During this same interview Greineder remained insistent that Mabel had given him a backrub that morning. Clearly the discovery of his

DNA beneath her fingernails was weighing heavily on his mind.

On November 3, Greineder was among the seven hundred mourners who packed Newton Presbyterian Church for a memorial service for Mabel. Through a friend he told the congregation: "The thread woven through May was her tremendous sense of responsibility to everyone. She needed to know that she made a difference to some person or some animal." (It was later learned that Greineder's fond memories of his wife didn't extend to collecting her ashes after she was cremated. They sat for six months in the funeral director's storage room, until Ilsa decided that enough was enough, and moved her sister's remains to the family vault in New York.)

As a proven liar, Greineder now started drawing even more heat. Twelve days after the crime the police returned to 56 Cleveland Road, armed with yet another search warrant. This time, in the garage, they found two self-prescribed bottles of Viagra that Greineder had obtained on April 3, 1998, and June 2, 1999, and a pack of Trojan condoms. Why, they wondered, would a husband purportedly press-ganged into a life of celibacy, stash a treasure trove of sexual goodies in the garage? Only one answer seemed to make any sense.

If Dirk Greineder was having an affair, then nobody close to the family had any inkling. Or if they did, they certainly weren't telling. Given the ruthless efficiency of most neighborhood grapevines, detectives doubted that Greineder could have kept any long-term liaison under wraps. They had him marked down as a one-nighter. It was now a case of putting Dirk Greineder's life under the microscope.

Modern technology is ruthlessly unforgiving. It can track our movements with laser-like precision and the footprints that we leave can be tracked for decades. Very few areas of modern life escape this intrusion—shopping receipts, phone records, cell phones themselves, credit cards, bank statements, personal computers—nothing is sacrosanct. Our reliance on these conveniences comes with a heavy price tag, as Greineder was just about to discover.

Cross referencing cell-phone records and credit card records revealed that, on February 8, 1998, Greineder had contacted the Commonwealth Entertainment escort agency, and that shortly thereafter a young woman named Elizabeth Porter arrived at the Crowne Plaza hotel in Natick, west of Boston. Greineder was waiting in a room filled with champagne, roses, chocolate-covered strawberries and assorted other fruit and candies. As they nibbled and quaffed, Greineder explained that he was a California-based doctor who frequently visited Boston for medical research. When Elizabeth pointed to his wedding band, he admitted being married, but said he was separated. His wife, he explained, had gone "soft," and there was no passion in the marriage. With his rationalizations and hors d'oevres out of the way, Greineder decided it was time for the main course. After the sex, Elizabeth Porter left.

Five days later, Greineder contacted Elizabeth again. This time they met at another Boston hotel. Greineder handed over $450 for a ninety-minute session that included him watching her as she took a shower, then massaging her with oil before they had sex. Elizabeth later said that this encounter left her feeling slightly uneasy, and although she admitted that she would have been ready for another assignation with the bizarre doctor, because she left the escort agency and changed her pager number, their paths never crossed again.

Further digging into Greineder's paperwork revealed his determination to keep as much of his secret life under wraps as possible. A clutch of credit cards bills were found for a shadowy firm called Physician's Consultants, a firm that seemed to exist nowhere else except in the imagination of Dirk Greineder. It turned out to be merely a vehicle for him to obtain two corporate credit cards from American Express. The cards were issued in July 1998 in the names of Greineder and someone called Thomas Young. Background checks showed that, while at Yale, Greineder had roomed with a Thomas Gorsuch Young III. When the police contacted Young, who lived in Glyndon, Maryland, the insurance company lawyer remembered Greineder well—"Very bright . . . and likeable"—but he struggled to recall their last meeting. A cocktail party in the mid-1960s, he thought. They hadn't spoken since 1969. After that, they'd exchanged Christmas cards for a couple years and then completely lost touch. So it came as something of a shock, to say the least, for Young to find that, thirty years later, his identity had been hijacked by his old college roommate in order to pay for romps in hotel rooms with high-priced call girls.

Henceforth, most of Greineder's sexual transactions were paid for with the Young credit card, and as the investigators tracked the paper trail left by the horny doctor, they stumbled across a possibly revealing coincidence. On June 2, 1999—the very day he wrote himself a prescription for Viagra—Greineder phoned yet another escort agency, and through them had sex with a young woman named Deborah Doolio at the Dedham Hilton. Doolio obviously pushed all the right buttons. In the days following this tryst, Greineder bombarded her with calls. During the course of these phone conversations, he often rambled, frantic in case his children found out about his double life. The calls turned into something of a miniconfessional, with Deborah donning her best counseling guise, telling

Greineder that he seemed "indecisive and . . . confused," and advising him that "seeing an escort wasn't the best thing for him to do until he found some peace within himself." In a thoughtful codicil, she demonstrated that her pecuniary interests hadn't been entirely sidetracked by confirming that she "would be available" if he needed her services at any time.

If Greineder heeded her advice, it didn't show. His sexual indiscretions took on new urgency, right up until a few days before Mabel's murder. On October 23, 1999, while attending a business conference, he stayed at the Sheraton Hotel in Mahwah, New Jersey. The adult movie he charged to his room at a cost of $16.95 obviously left him hungry for more, because hotel records log him trawling the Internet until the early hours. At 3 AM he found what he was after—a local escort agency. A quick dash to the ATM in the lobby, and he was raring to go when the object of his attentions showed at four o'clock. For a guy pushing sixty, Greineder obviously had plenty of stamina. Just a few hours after the young woman left at 6 AM, he was on the lecture podium, looking as fresh as a daisy. Later that day he returned to the family fold at Wellesley.

While at home, like most modern academics, Greineder relied heavily on his computer. It proved invaluable in his research work, it allowed him to footnote his wife's term paper—the hard drive showed that the document had last been saved at 12:12 AM, just eight hours before she was murdered—and it provided yet another conduit for Greineder's sexual cravings. What he failed to appreciate was that his progress was being monitored every step of the way.

Even supposedly sophisticated computer users can display a quite staggering level of ignorance when it comes to their use. For instance, in 1997, when veteran British glam-rocker Gary Glitter decided to bring his computer into a shop for repair, he did so without once imagining that anyone would find the reams of pedophiliac images he had downloaded from the Internet. A technician, shocked and sickened by the nauseating pictures, wasted no time in contacting the police. Glitter's oversight or arrogance, call it what you will, ultimately led to public disgrace, a prison sentence, followed by self-imposed exile abroad.* Fortunately such foolishness is rife in the criminal community; as the Harvard-based doctor was about to find out.

For Greineder, the computer was far more than a mere work tool, it was his gateway into the dark, often dangerous world of Internet adult chatrooms. Here, surfing anonymously—or so he thought—he was free to swap fantasies and arrange assignations with other like-minded individuals. In one of his breathy communications he leered, "I think that I have dabbled with almost anything you can think of, though my preferences remain pretty vanilla (if you call threesomes vanilla!!)."

Another woman with whom he exchanged e-mails was told, "Loved your pics! Looks like you are into some [bondage and domination] too. I have some interest/experience with this though I have given up all of my toys. Maybe you still have some! But mostly, I liked the images and I am sure that I will love to play with you."

Greineder's online urgency peaked just one week before his wife's murder, as he fired off a torrent of e-mails to various sex-related websites. Calling himself "CasualGuy200," he contacted one couple through an online dating agency, tapping out his fantasies on the keyboard: "I am white, married, but she does not play. So I'm looking for a very discreet

*Upon his release, Glitter fled abroad. In 2006 he was convicted in Vietnam for molesting underage girls and jailed for another three years.

couple with whom to play. I also am very oral, both give and receive and would love to exchange e-mails to see if we can fit. I am a few pounds overweight, really only a few. Love group activities. I am basically straight, but can be flexible in group situations." As a teaser, Greineder attached a full frontal nude photograph of himself. It failed to impress and no threesome was arranged.

In the wake of this abortive attempt at cyber-dating, October 30 saw Greineder again phoning Deborah Doolio and leaving a message on her voice mail. She didn't reply. What effect this had on his psyche we don't know. What is certain is that just hours later Mabel Greineder was bludgeoned and butchered at Morse's Pond. That night, as the newly bereaved widower sat alone in his house, it was Deborah again to whom he attempted to turn. His luck hadn't improved; she still didn't get back to him.

With his private life stripped bare, Greineder gave the investigators what they were looking for: a motive for killing his wife. They speculated—and that is all it ever amounted to, speculation—that somehow Mabel had found out about her husband's nocturnal ramblings and threatened him with public exposure. Greineder, fearing ruination, had then battered and slashed her to death. If this scenario was accurate, then clearly Mabel's indignation did not extend to forgoing the customary morning walk with her errant husband. Perhaps she was hoping to patch things up? Perhaps, the prosecutors had it all wrong? Certainly people who'd known Mabel all her life took the view that she was the kind of person prepared to sweep any scandal—no matter how hurtful—under the carpet rather than jeopardize her children's well-being. With Kirsten's wedding just around the corner, the last thing on Mabel's mind would have been blowing the whistle on Dirk's philandering.

Such reasoning didn't deflect the Commonwealth of

Massachusetts. It took four months and nine search warrants to build their case, but on February 29, 2000, Dr. Dirk Greineder was arrested at his Brookline office and charged with his wife's murder. Apart from his three children, nobody could claim to be shocked. The only surprise had been the amount of time it took the state to file charges. It was a tardiness born of circumspection—they feared a repetition of the Burke fiasco. Greineder, they knew, would be able to afford legal representation of the highest caliber; any hint of prosecutorial overzealousness and the defense would be jumping all over them.

The indignities piled up around the disgraced doctor. One week after being taken into custody, he heard that his license to practice medicine had been suspended. The state medical board had deemed him to be a threat to public health and safety.

This was a truly miserable time for Massachusetts medicine. Just four months after Greineder was arrested, another local physician was making headlines for all the wrong reasons. On July 14, 2000, Dr. Richard Sharpe, a cross-dressing millionaire dermatologist with a fondness for prescription drugs, chose to sidestep the tedium of an expensive and messy divorce by shooting his wife through the chest at the family home in Wenham, just northeast of Boston. (After an interstate chase, Sharpe was captured the next day and later sentenced to life imprisonment.)

Yet another hammer blow to the Hippocratic Oath in Massachusetts was delivered less than a week after Sharpe gunned down his wife. This came when Dr. James Kartell was convicted of slaying his wife's lover, Janos Vajda, two years earlier at a hospital in Methuen. Found guilty of involuntary manslaughter, Kartell received five to eight years in prison.

But it was the Greineder case that made the biggest

headlines of all, fueled in no small part by the state's seeming determination to leak every single detail of the doctor's colorful sex life to a salivating media. In some ways this proved counterproductive. First, it allowed breast-beating defense attorneys to thunder that their client was being tried in the media; second, it allowed them to throw a useful smokescreen around what had become an almost unanswerable forensic case against the accused.

At its heart were the two Ziploc storage bags found close to the crime scene. These had been sent for analysis to Lorie Gottesman, a documents and plastics expert at the FBI crime lab. Storage bags are made from huge sheets of melted plastic that pass over rollers. Part of the manufacturing process calls for a blade to make the perforations that enable the bags to be ripped from the end of the roll; elsewhere on the production line, a heat seal melts the bottom of the bag and seals it tightly. With millions of feet of plastic being processed daily comes an inevitable buildup of debris on the heat seal, thus ensuring that, while bags made within seconds of each other are microscopically similar, bags made at either end of the working day will display markedly different heat-seal characteristics. When compared microscopically, the two bags found at the crime scene displayed the same striations as the seven found in Greineder's kitchen, leading Gottesman to conclude that the bags were made within seconds of each other. To all intents and purposes, they were identical.

More damning evidence—a cash register receipt—had been found in Greineder's workshop. He was a keen home handyman, and this receipt showed that on September 3, 1999, he had purchased $6.76 worth of nails at his local hardware store, F. Diehl & Sons. A check of Diehl's register tapes disclosed that just three minutes after Greineder had bought the nails, someone paid $31.49 for an Estwing drill hammer—a miniature sledgehammer identical to the one used to bludgeon Mabel six weeks later. While no one at the store that day could positively identify Greineder as the person who had bought both items, the fact that the two transactions were sequential and that Diehl's records showed this to be the only Estwing drill hammer they sold that month, made for powerful circumstantial evidence.

Diehl & Sons again figured prominently when Trooper Foley went looking for a match for the distinctive brown Librett gloves with their rubber-textured palm and fingers. Of the nearly thirty stores that he checked, only Diehl & Sons had them in stock.

And then there was the DNA evidence. It had been analyzed by Dr. Robin Cotton of Cellmark Diagnostics, a hardnosed scientist, well used to the rough and tumble of courtroom testimony, having spent five days on the stand during the O. J. Simpson trial. Her tests on DNA recovered from the right-hand brown work glove found alongside the knife, matched eight of thirteen determining points in the complicated testing procedure used to give a profile. She calculated the chances of this DNA coming from someone other than Dirk Greineder at one in 170 million. Traces of Greineder's DNA were also detected on the left-hand glove found a few yards from his parked van. This yielded seven of nine determining points. Cotton concluded that only one in 680,000 Caucasians could match that profile. She was appropriately circumspect when it came to the four-inch folding knife. All she would say was that she could not exclude Dirk Greineder as being a secondary source of DNA found on the handle.

Cotton had also located two tiny drops of blood on the small red backpack that Greineder had been seen wearing on the day of the murder. A mixture of DNA extracted from the blood showed the primary source as being Mabel

Greineder, prompting speculation that Greineder had used the backpack to transport the bloody weapons to their hiding place after the murderous attack.

As often happens in many criminal cases, it was the negative evidence that spoke loudest of all. On the day of the attack, Greineder insisted that when he found his stricken wife he had checked for a pulse in her bloody neck. That same day he consented when, in a routine procedure, investigators requested a sample of his fingernail clippings. Yet when Cotton tested these clippings, she could not find anyone else's DNA present except that of Dirk Greineder. This absence of foreign DNA further strengthened the state's belief that Greineder had worn the brown work gloves during the attack, and that at no time had he checked for a pulse in Mabel's neck, as he had claimed.

Given all the lurid pretrial publicity, the defense had high hopes that their request for a change of venue would receive a sympathetic hearing from the bench, but in the end Judge Paul Chernoff decided that the trial would be held in Dedham. So it was that on May 23, 2001, Dr. Dirk Greineder finally got to face his accusers in the same courthouse where eight decades earlier Sacco and Vanzetti had been catapulted into left-wing martyrdom.

The trial followed a predictable path, with the prosecution portraying Greineder as a sexual obsessive, someone prepared to kill the woman he had lived with for thirty-one years rather than face the ignominy of public exposure. His cynicism, they claimed, was breathtaking. He had exploited the local hysteria surrounding recent events in Norfolk County and butchered his wife in cold blood, hoping to pass off her murder as just one in a string of serial killings.

No, no, no, replied the defense, here was a man who had strayed and paid mightily for his errant ways, but he remained a loving husband and a devoted father. Blinkered investigative prejudice had victimized an innocent man and brought him to this court today. Within hours of the murder, the police had rushed to judgment, decided that Greineder was the killer, and refused to consider any other possibility. Why on earth would a renowned allergist with a PhD in pharmacology take his wife to a public spot if he intended to kill her? Surely if he really wanted to get rid of Mabel, it would be child's play for him to administer an untraceable drug in the seclusion and safety of his own home? This may have sounded superficially plausible, but as we have already seen with Coppolino and Friedgood, access to almost untraceable poisons is no guarantee of success. Besides, what better disguise for a sophisticated physician to adopt than that of the frenzied butcher?

None of the defense arguments could deflect the barrage of direct and circumstantial evidence that all pointed toward Dirk Greineder as the killer. And that was without factoring in the testimony of the numerous prostitutes and online "swingers" who provided titillating insights into the defendant's ravenous sexual appetites. Faced by such an onslaught, it is hardly surprising that Greineder took the nowadays somewhat unusual step of testifying on his own behalf. Looking gaunt from his time behind bars and ghostly pale, he was on the stand for three days. He sobbed, he admitted his failings, saying that sexual frustration had driven him reluctantly into the arms of prostitutes only as a last resort, but, most of all, he proclaimed his undying love for Mabel. When it came to cross-examination he seemed less assured and far more willful. Suddenly the contradictions began to appear, then the excuses, then the look of bewildered guilt. In the end, the only surprise was that it took the jury four days to reach their decision.

On June 29, 2001, when the guilty verdict was delivered, Greineder bowed his head and grimaced. The sentence was the only one allowable for first-degree murder under Massachusetts law: life imprisonment without the possibility of parole. He turned and said good-bye to his three children, who stood holding hands as they watched their father disappear. He continues to appeal his conviction and sentence, but the latest setback came on May 9, 2006, when his request for a retrial was denied.

So far as the forensic evidence told against Greineder, it was a slam dunk. Once again, a doctor had tried to defeat the legal system and failed. Although it was never proved, there is strong reason to suspect that the prosecution got the motive right: Greineder killed his wife because she had discovered his secret life, and threatened him with public exposure. Nothing else seems to make sense. After all, years of alleged sexual abstinence had first been endured and then accommodated with a string of prostitutes, and then suddenly, out of the blue, he reaches for the hammer and the knife. On one level the utter amateurishness of the operation suggests a spur-of-the-moment madness, yet no one can doubt that this was a carefully planned execution. When Dirk Greineder left home that morning, he did so fully intending that his wife should die within the hour. He'd stashed a kit of murder tools in his backpack, he led his victim to a deserted part of the woods where he hammered and slashed her to death, and he attempted to blame his actions on another phantom killer. Crimes don't come much more premeditated.*

In the space of sixteen months, three Massachusetts physicians were charged with murdering their wives. All

*Checks on a DNA database subsequently led investigators to arrest a convicted murderer named Martin Guy for the murder of Irene Kennedy. He was convicted of this crime on September 27, 2006, and sentenced to life without parole.

were caught and all were convicted, proof that when passion gets the better of brains, then all the qualifications in the world won't come to your rescue. But perhaps there was something else at work here, an overweening arrogance that the chief prosecutor, Richard Grundy, touched upon in his closing argument to the Greineder jury: "The defendant's greatest defense here is that you don't want to believe that an upstanding physician in an upstanding profession . . . could commit such a crime."

Unwittingly, perhaps, but with these words, Grundy could well have been describing any of the killer doctors in this book.

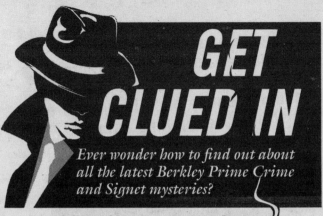

Don't miss the page-turning suspense, intriguing characters, and unstoppable action that keep readers coming back for more from these bestselling authors...

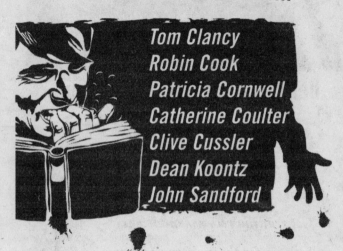

Tom Clancy
Robin Cook
Patricia Cornwell
Catherine Coulter
Clive Cussler
Dean Koontz
John Sandford

Your favorite thrillers and suspense novels come from Berkley.

penguin.com